The Mosaic of Care

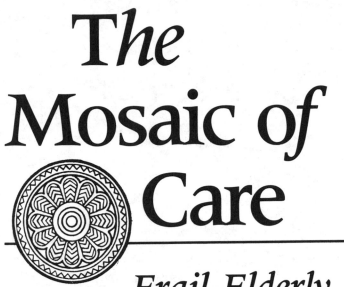

*Frail Elderly
and Their Families
in the Real World*

The
Mosaic of
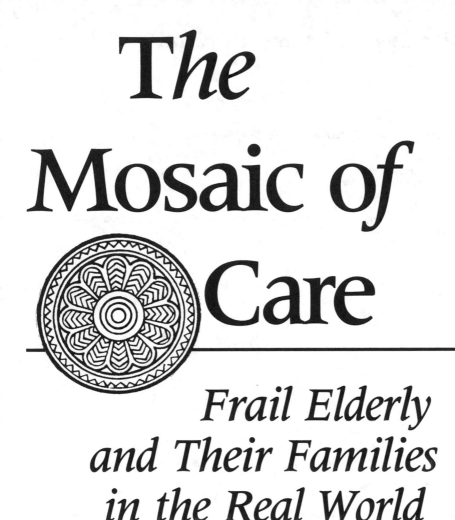
Care

*Frail Elderly
and Their Families
in the Real World*

Jaber F. Gubrium

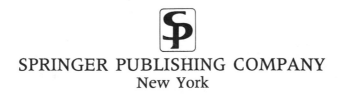

SPRINGER PUBLISHING COMPANY
New York

For Eva and Albert Olweean

Library of Congress Cataloging-in-Publication Data

Gubrium, Jaber F.
  The mosaic of care: frail elderly and their families in the real world/Jaber F. Gubrium.
    p.   cm.
  Includes bibliographical references.
  ISBN 0-8261-7570-8
    1. Frail elderly—Care—United States.   2. Frail elderly—United States—
  Family relationships.   I. Title.
  HV1461.G83   1990
362.6—dc20   90-35878
                                                                        CIP

Published by Springer Publishing Co.

Printed in the United States of America.

Contents

Preface

Running through the popular and professional literature of frail elderly and their families is an image of impairment, caregiving burdens, and nursing homes. The image presents frail elderly concerned with "brain failure," decreasing mobility, and hopelessness, among a wide-range of debilitating conditions. Families are portrayed as insufferably plagued by "36-hour days" of care and monitoring, the guilt of nursing home placement, and attempts to readjust their lives afterward. The picture is one of gloom and doom. While overtures are made to potentially positive conditions such as the availability of social support for family caregivers, the absence of support is interpreted to have undesirable, if not dire, consequences for all concerned.

Images, of course, contain grains of truth. As persons age, they are likely to experience concomitant impairments and face the portent of being incapacitated. Not uncommon are falls and fractured hips, heart failure, strokes, and forgetfulness. Families can, and many do, become stressed in the care of elderly members.

Are these the signal themes of care and caregiving for elderly? When we ask what the conditions and responses *mean* to those concerned, we discover a much more complicated picture. There are alternate, contradictory, interpenetrating, and shifting truths. Stories of the terrible trouble resulting from lapses of memory contrast with entirely benign versions of the same occurrences. Tales of tribulation regarding the sudden strain of caring for an increasingly demented spouse are strikingly different from the total commitment that makes light of caregiving's relatively minor inconveniences. Such are the differences in what commonly is called "the real world," where stories and versions of caregiving events and conditions engage us in the experience of diversity.

In 20 years of ethnographic research in aging, I never have ceased to be amazed by the vibrant variation in people's experiences of growing older. In tracing the many conditions and contexts that shape lives, it is evident that the way lives are put together cannot be reduced to a collection of facts, statistical correlates, or formal explanatory models. There are too many styles of living and coping, manifold circumstances, points of view, interests, and loose ends to be accommodated by a metric.

The Mosaic of Care is written for professional service workers—nurses, family physicians, psychiatrists, psychologists, social workers, case managers, pastoral counselors, health care administrators, and therapists—offering a way to understand diversity in the lives of frail elderly and their families. Its stories and interpretations are also directly relevant to the broader audience of all who, day in and day out, encounter the frailties of old age, including family caregivers themselves. They will recognize that in the real world the problems of aging are not simple and straightforward but are more or less trouble according to the caregivers' ties and interpersonal traditions with those cared for.

The book's central questions are: How are the lives of frail elderly and their families organized in the real world and how can knowledge of this organization inform professional caregivers? The book aims to fill the gap between what professionals are taught in the classroom and what can be learned from a careful examination of practice, encouraging them to accept and address the real world in its own terms, not exclusively in terms of theory. While the book offers a new beginning for professionally approaching frail elderly and their families, it also envisions a new gerontology, emphasizing the interpretive complications of ordinary experience.

The stories presented are taken from real life, located in the numerous settings where I conducted fieldwork, from the community to the nursing home (see Appendix). The names of persons and places have been changed to protect their identities. The stories and versions are not a statistically random sample of the general population of frail elderly, their families, and service providers, nor of the settings and circumstances that contain their lives. The selection has a different purpose: to represent the diverse and complex interpretations of aging, frailty, and its cares.

Although the idea of a linear continuum of care is questioned, it nonetheless serves to organize the presentation. The first chapter lays the conceptual groundwork. The reader then is introduced to stories showing the social complications of frail elderly lives in the context of a range of settings and caregiving considerations. The concluding chapter builds on the stories to conceptualize intervention in the real world.

A much ignored feature of the real world is that knowledge of it comes in the form of stories—ordinary narratives and tales of joy and woe about ourselves and others. These are the essential stuff of *The Mosaic of Care*, presented according to the ways those who make their lives in the real world articulate and act upon them.

J.F.G.
Gainesville, Florida
April, 1990

Acknowledgments

I take this opportunity to acknowledge those who have, over the years, either directly or indirectly influenced my interpretation of the aging experience and caregiving. The research and writing of two gerontologists and a medical sociologist have been important in general: Bernice Neugarten's insistent probing into the kinds of experience that growing older can be; David Gutmann's creative cross-cultural attempt to trace the themes and variations of later life among men and women; and Anselm Strauss's outstanding analyses of the contexts of caregiving and care receiving. Recently, I have been much intrigued by the work of several anthropologists who have, as is their delightful habit, shown us, and me, the intricacies of the meaning of care: Colleen Johnson, Sharon Kaufman, Jennie Keith, Mark Luborsky, Linda Mitteness, Robert Rubinstein, and Andrea Sankar. The insights of Emily Abel, Ann Dill, Lucy Fischer, Myrna Silverman, and Clare Wenger also have been useful. Their collective influence resonates in the chapters of this book.

I owe a special debt of gratitude to Victoria Bumagin, who first mentioned to me the idea of turning ethnography into something useful to the professional caregiver. She invited me to speak to a group of professionals and interested laypersons as part of the Center for Applied Gerontology's lecture program in Chicago. It was such a warm reception that I eventually made good on the idea at the behest of Jean Lesher, my supportive editor. It is now my firm belief that we academics have an obligation to speak to those we study and the public at large.

My approach to aging is part of a general orientation to the study of experience, emphasizing interpretation, social ties, and context. This has centered recently on life stories, especially their social construction, varied meanings, and organizational embeddedness. I thank the following friends for helping me to clarify the place of communication and narrative in everyday life: David Buckholdt, Robert Dingwall, James Holstein, Gale Miller, and David Silverman.

A number of colleagues read *The Mosaic of Care* in manuscript and commented on it: R. Satyanarayana, Abraham Monk, Robert Rubinstein, Margaret Hellie Huyck, and Terrie Wetle. I appreciate their many suggestions.

I have come to realize how much bearing the good common sense of my wife, Suzanne, has had on my writing. More than anyone, she urges me to write for the general reader, whose native intelligence she repeatedly warns me never to doubt. I have tried to take her advice into account in writing this book and am pleased to have done so.

The
Mosaic of
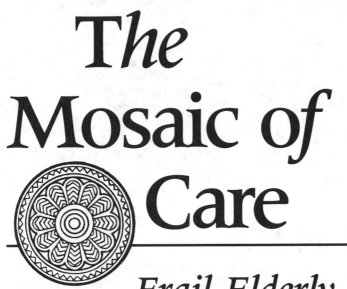 # Care

*Frail Elderly
and Their Families
in the Real World*

CHAPTER 1

"Welcome to the Real World!"

The Incident

According to a very visible clique of elderly women on the residential floor of a nursing home, another elderly resident, John, had "absolutely lost all his marbles" and, besides, was the vilest man alive. The women complained that John repeatedly used "their" bathing room (bathroom), located at "their" end of the corridor, when he just as easily could have used the one near his own room. While the bathrooms served the personal care needs of all residents, those whose own rooms were located in the vicinity of one tended to claim it as their own. As clique members were in the habit of loudly musing, "Why anyone would want to come over here to take a bath when he could use the bathroom at the other end is beyond me."

An "outrageous" incident brought the matter to a head, proving John's demented status to the clique. One of the women, Lillian, had been using the bathroom in the clique's area. The women had agreed to post a sign on the bathroom door when it was occupied to "prevent the likes of John from mistakenly walking in and setting his dirty eyes on everything and everyone." While none admittedly saw what happened, the incident was vividly detailed, as if all had actually been there.

THE WOMEN'S VIEW

The women reported that things were pretty quiet that morning until they started to put "two and two together," as several mentioned. Bella believed she had seen John walking along with his cane but guessed that he was doing the usual, which was "gadding about" at their end of the hallway where he "really has no business," instead of at the other end. Since the women were habitually in their rooms after breakfast, Bella thought little of John's presence. After all, she explained later, he might simply be taking his morning constitutional, as others did on the floor. Another woman thought she'd heard someone say, "Get out," but dismissed it as coming from one of the several, barely audible nearby television sets.

Suddenly there was a chilling scream, "like someone was being murdered in cold blood," one of the women observed. Several remarked that it nearly frightened them to death. None wanted to look into what was happening. Each explained how she felt frozen to her chair or bed. A few minutes later, Phoebe, a vocal leader of the group, stuck her head out the doorway of her room, looking down the hall. While the screaming seemed to come from that direction, there was no one to be seen. But, then, as chilling as before, yet clearer, she heard, "Get out of here, John! Get out!" Phoebe recognized the voice immediately. It was that of her dear friend, Lillian. She heard John, too, unmistakably shout back, "Shut up, you old bag! This room isn't your property! I can come in here any time I want. You old bags think you own the place!"

Phoebe reported later that she really wanted to help, but she felt all she could do was to yell that John was hurting Lillian. After what seemed to be an eternity, John walked out of the bathroom waving his cane, caught it in the handrail along the hallway, and stumbled. According to the women, that was to be expected when the devil was at work, and it served John right. What's more, they felt that if the fall incapacitated John, maybe he'd be transferred to one of the patient floors where care requirements were higher and where the staff was prepared to handle the demented.

The story of the incident was told and retold by the women. Each embellished it according to the part she construed herself as playing. Whether because Phoebe was a vocal leader or because of the crucial part she claimed to have in the incident, her version was the most widely conveyed. It was a blow-by-blow account of an occurrence that, in retrospect, "was bound to happen." Indeed, as Phoebe quickly reported to the nursing home's social worker, Miss Hanson, "I just knew that John was going to walk in there someday while someone was taking a bath, and I had a sneaking suspicion that it was going to be real soon." Phoebe explained further that all the women on the floor knew John was *non compos mentis* and really, really rude, dirty-minded, and foul-mouthed on top of it." She pointed out that if she hadn't bothered to yell, John probably would have stayed in the bathroom all morning, that he might have "even raped Lillian or given her a heart attack." As the self-appointed representative of the women on the floor, Phoebe demanded that for safety's sake Miss Hanson "do something about John and do it quick!"

Phoebe's was not the only complaint filed with Miss Hanson. Two other clique members described the incident as a frightening occurrence that now continues to "go through [their] minds." As Hazel reported, she had been lying on her bed taking a short nap when she heard the yelling and screaming. She didn't know who it was or what it was all about, but "it sure sounded bloodcurdling." What went through her mind at the time was that she wasn't sure if she was awake or dreaming. When she heard Phoebe yell, she opened her eyes but dared not move from her bed. Hazel then put "two and two together" and thought that John actually must be causing real harm, not just being a pest. As Hazel complained to Miss Hanson, "I just can't keep myself calm anymore. It's caused me such a fright, and I worry all the time that maybe I'll be the next one."

Another clique member, Velma, told Hanson that she was knitting and watching a game show on television when she heard the scuffle. She knew Lillian was in the bathroom because Lillian had stopped by earlier to borrow some powder Velma had recommended. But Velma explained that she didn't put "two and two together" until much later, not until Phoebe came into her room to report that John was at it again. Even then, Velma couldn't believe John would do such a thing—walk into a room while a lady was taking her bath. It was unconscionable. Becoming teary-eyed as she complained to Miss Hanson, it was just one more of a series of incidents that made Velma feel completely unsafe. As she cried, "Today, people have just lost all sense of the rules, and I'm afraid it's no different in here than on the streets." According to Velma, the question that now kept going through her mind was: "What is becoming of the world?"

A NURSE'S VIEW

Shortly thereafter, when Miss Hanson spoke to the licensed practical nurse (LPN) temporarily on duty the morning of the incident, things took on a different tone. The LPN was not altogether pleased that she now was responsible for writing a formal incident report because John had stumbled and bruised his shoulder. It was one more task, among others, that made her job difficult. Not only are "unreasonable demands" made on her time from the residents, but what with their constant bickering, the general intolerance, and the possessiveness, "it's a wonder that they're not actually at each other's throats," she commented.

While the LPN was acquainted with the diverse social ties and sentiments of the floor, the incident report form merely required a description of John's mental status at the time of the incident and the events leading up to it. When Hanson asked the LPN what she thought of John's mental status, the LPN observed, "John's the type of man, like some of his friends, that I think sometimes has a confused set of values." When Hanson commented that she had had complaints that John was too confused to remain on the residential floor, the LPN remarked that John could confuse everyone with all his conniving, adding, "And sometimes it backfires on him, like the fall he took." (Evidently, Hanson and the LPN accorded different meanings to confusion.)

At lunch the next day, Miss Hanson heard another slant on the incident from the same LPN, this time decidedly comical. Part of the general gossip and folklore about patients and residents, staff members regularly recounted "really amusing" moments of life in the nursing home. The bathroom incident seemed to be the latest. According to the LPN, John had made a fool of himself scaring Phoebe's uppity group half to death when he virtually exposed himself in one of the first-floor bathrooms. As the LPN explained, John had been pretty angry the whole week because he'd been repeatedly harassed by the group. Whenever John passed them in the hallway or in the lobby, they made a point of turning their heads and scattering about like frightened hens. Clique members also would whisper loud enough for John to hear them say that he had lost all his marbles and should be transferred to a skilled-care floor. The LPN explained that when she overheard John accusing them of talking behind his back, they denied they had said anything at all and asserted that John was hearing things as usual and should get his ears examined.

WHAT MISS HANSON PIECED TOGETHER

Miss Hanson knew that the sniping between John, his friends, and Phoebe's clique had gotten particularly bad. What happened that morning was part of a history of mutual resentment and competition for status. Still, as one of those gathered at lunch pointed out, there was good and bad in both groups. Phoebe's clique could be considerate and gracious, showering staff and others with small favors. The clique also could be cruel to those they resented, John among them. John's collection of friends, too, had its good and bad sides. John was the floor's most riotous, if not ribald, storyteller. Staff were regularly amused by his good humor, quick wit, and intriguing tales, sharing many themselves. Yet, John was no respecter of social airs; they offended him deeply.

Combining these qualities, a different version of the bathroom incident developed, liberally sprinkled with mockery. Miss Hanson heard about a confrontation between John, Lillian, and others that was more slapstick than sober. John became the proverbial sly fox with an eye for the women. Lillian took on the demeanor of a demure lady. Phoebe was the protective witch. In this version, the incident was a parody on the confrontation of purity and danger, in which all played appropriate and recognizable black-and-white roles. It was a medley of clowns, in which the residents were more characters toying with appearances than clashing personalities. Embarrassment was something to laugh about, not a lesson about the invasion of privacy. Anger was more amusing than it was a point of sympathetic resentment. The climax of this telling was conveyed in terms of "what *must* have gone through their minds" when Lillian saw John peek at her in the bathtub. One staff member remarked that he would have given anything to see the expressions on their faces. The question of whether John actually "peeked" at Lillian or Lillian actually saw John in the bathroom did not spoil what was otherwise a thoroughly enjoyable drama about "things that happen in a place like this."

JOHN AND HIS FRIENDS' VIEW

When Miss Hanson spoke to John and a few of his friends, the happenings of that fateful morning were less an incident than a coup. According to the friends, the unfortunate thing about it was that John got a bit "roughed up" in the process, not that he caused fear and trembling among some of the residents. Indeed, a comparison of their version of what happened with what Hanson heard from Phoebe raised the question in Hanson's mind of whether she had heard the same events described.

One of John's friends noted that they had been talking for a long time about the "old bags" down the hall and what should be done about their bossiness and claims on "everything in this place." Another friend, Sadie, joked about how the men had decided to give clique members "the old hiss-hiss routine," which entailed hissing loudly as members passed nearby. But according to John, "The straw that broke the camel's back was when I walked into that bathroom and pretended that I didn't know where I was." John pointed out that he knew "just about when they liked to take a bath in there." On the morning of the incident, he guessed that he'd just stroll down the hall to see what was happening. Sadie interjected jovially, "Yeah and we all knew what you were up to, John. Don't give us that innocent act." John chuckled. The telling seemed to be as much fun as the events reported.

John described how he had found no one in the vicinity of the bathroom. Several nearby doors were closed or slightly ajar. He recounted how he "made [his] move," as he put it, pushing open the bathroom door and slipping inside without knocking his cane against anything. Inside, he wasn't sure who was using the facilities, but was almost certain it was one of the "old bags." Before John continued with the story, he mused, "I wish it was old Phoebe, but it didn't matter that much because they'd all get mad as hell anyway." John explained how he acted surprised to hear that he wasn't alone in the bathroom and how he had innocently remarked that he had mistaken the bathroom door for a different one. When he was told to get out of the bathroom, he hesitated until he was screamed at by a woman he later gathered was Lillian. At that point, John reported that he quickly left the bathroom. On his way out, he stumbled a bit, but immediately pulled himself together and walked away. John concluded, "I'll never know why that girl [the LPN] made such a big stink about that little slip, making a report and all that stuff."

FAMILY INVOLVEMENT

Miss Hanson soon heard complaints about the incident from residents' families. Phoebe's son, for one, had spoken to the administrator of the nursing home about the lack of privacy in the facility. The administrator conveyed the concern to Hanson and asked her to check into the problem. In related communications, other staff members reported that they had been told in no uncertain terms by family members that it was their understanding that the first floor of the nursing home was residential, limited to elderly persons only in need of personal care, and no place for the demented, confused, or otherwise incapacitated. Much of what Hanson heard directly and indirectly from family members supported the view that John was mentally unfit to remain in the residential unit.

When Hanson presented John's case to the staff members in a patient care conference, she attempted to convey each side of the story. She indicated that while she was trying to be fair to both Phoebe's and John's group, the home also had to think about families' concerns in the matter, especially in view of the fact that Phoebe's son had warned the administrator that several families would "pull" their residents out of the home and "give it a bad name" if things weren't changed. The social worker concluded, "It's not a very pretty picture. Whatever we do will be unfair to someone." Before anything more was said, the associate director of nursing announced, "Welcome to the real world!"

The Real World

This expression by the associate director of nursing, no doubt, is familiar to most. In two decades of ethnographic fieldwork in human service institutions and community care settings studying frail elderly and their families, I have heard it and similar statements many times.

DIRECT REFERENCES

Occasionally, it comes in the form of a precaution to professional workers in training. For example, occupational therapy (OT) interns in a rehabilitation hospital studied in the late seventies (Gubrium & Buckholdt, 1982) often are told to "wait until you get into the real world," as they now and then question interpretations of physical assessments. It is not uncommon for the OT interns themselves to compare what they are learning in school with hospital practice. While the interns have been taught, say, how to assess objectively the full range of motion of the upper extremities, they find that the hospital's practicing OTs take into consideration the family's expectations for recovery in figuring the measures. The interns' training leaves such social contingencies out of the picture, or allocates them to a miscellaneous category of "other" factors.

It is not that the OT interns have been taught improperly nor that the quality of occupational therapy in this hospital is poor. By conventional standards, both are well above average. Indeed, in relation to the real world of practice inside the hospital, interns are sometimes cautioned that they have to unlearn or rethink some of what they have learned too well. This is a serious matter. Interns know that the hospital is not to be glibly dismissed, since it has a formidable reputation as a specialized treatment center. The interns discover that, quality of care aside, the hospital's real world is set apart from the hospital world taken for granted in their formal training.

I also have heard references to the real world among more seasoned professionals. In the story above, the associate director of nursing's reference to "the real world" is a reminder that human service in theory does not automatically align with practice. This does not necessarily cast aspersion on practice in comparison with the ideal. As the associate director comments later, part of staff's "problem" is that Hanson bothered to investigate all sides of the incident and inadvertently showed how its events are understandable from several perspectives.

In contrast to the ideal, the real world is comprised of the full range of professional competencies and care qualities. The real world is peopled by ineffective OTs, physical therapists, social workers, physicians, and nurses as well as their effective counterparts. The real world contains both disgraceful treatment facilities and programs and stellar organizations and offerings. As it is put in the various field settings, in the real world "you find all kinds." In this regard, it should be added that a world completely filled with incompetent professionals and poor quality programs is as "unreal" as a world comprised of their opposites. The term *real world* does not as much pertain to the bad side of professional caregiving as it highlights its multifaceted conditions.

The difference between the ideal and the real is significant. The real world binds together contrasts and complications that are an integral part of the work of professional practice, which means that the features cannot be eliminated, only accommodated. The real world, after all, is "real," not to be wished away. The real world is the implicit background of forewarnings and announcements about the hard facts of life. While some long for the ideal world of text, theory, planning, and goal specification, all know that the real world, at the same time, is something one has "to live with." Those who feel they have become "hardened" believe the real world to be the only world of human service, the ideal being a world of fantasy. Whatever their thinking on the relation between real and ideal, a sense of the real world's obdurate and ineluctable character keeps all constantly attuned to it.

INDIRECT REFERENCES

There are other, less direct references. For example, physicians habitually distinguish the science and art of medicine. A geriatrician serving as a consultant to an Alzheimer's disease day care program studied in the mid-eighties (Gubrium, 1986a) regularly speaks of the significance of the "art" of medicine in persuading the families of Alzheimer's patients to start thinking about the family's well-being as much as about cure. The geriatrician observes that the aura that comes with being a doctor is as important an ingredient of medical effectiveness as his or her formal skills as a highly trained professional. He regularly reminds his staff that their training can take them "just so far" and that what it takes to be successful in the real world is handy, careful, and frequent attention to its peculiar demands. As the geriatrician advises, "You have to make a habit of it; make it a regular part of your work with families and patients."

Another indirect reference comes with the use of the terms "practice" and "practical." Professional workers routinely speak of how practice can be quite different from theory. It is not uncommon to hear them refer to what should happen in theory as opposed to what occurs in practice. While professionals use the term "theory" rather loosely, it nonetheless marks the border between what ideally should occur and what occurs in fact. Used in this way, the term "fact" pertains to facts of experience—to practice—not to the ideal facts of the scientific world (Raffel, 1979).

TWO SETS OF TERMS

In sum, two sets of terms specify different, yet equally important domains of understanding regarding caregiving. One domain is referenced by science, theory, and the ideal. The other domain is circumscribed by art, practice, and the real. Professional workers have extensive, formal knowledge of the first domain, derived from textbooks, classrooms, and professional literatures. The second domain, relegated to the art of their respective skills, is located in practice.

While all professional caregivers, from novices to veterans, recognize the meaning of these references to the real world and become adept at using their distinguishing terms, none of them has been formally prepared to deal with the distinction. What they have learned in training are fine skills, but skills both taught and received "in theory." While the best of them have learned the most advanced techniques and their varied applications, their formal acquaintance with the real world has been limited to internships, practicums, and field placements.

The wisdom gained from training placements in the real world comes in the form of narrative—complaints, anecdotes, tales of woe, gossip, accounts, atrocity stories, and folklore. It is a different kind of knowledge, with its own vocabulary and operational logic, about a world that resists the systematic and precise language of what is taught in theory.

Troubles, Ties, and Traditions

The real world is not just a handy way of referring to practice, but is socially organized. Three interpersonal features of the real world shape its stories: people's *troubles*, their *ties*, and their *traditions*.

TROUBLES

In practice, any problem such as a disease, care need, or physical dysfunction can trouble those concerned in different ways. In other words, any one problem is a configuration of separate troubles, depending on the point of view. I use the term "trouble" as the real-world counterpart of problem (Emerson & Messenger, 1977). In the bathroom incident, John's "problem" troubles him, Phoebe, Lillian, Sadie, the staff, and others differently. The troubles that, say, John's mental status pose are not necessarily consistent with each other in meaning or sentiment.

In theory, the nurses, doctors, social workers, and other health care providers in the field sites deal with problems such as diseases and care needs. Some are prepared to apply skills to alleviate bodily ailments such as diabetes, hip fractures, amputations, incontinence, and bed sores. Some deal with behavioral or mental problems, including depression, disorientation, confusion, and dementia. Others identify problems in activities of daily living or in physical functioning and offer their brands of treatment.

In the real world, diseases, care needs, and dysfunctions are not that straightforward. They are entangled with all kinds of other considerations—historical, interpersonal, and circumstantial. Take, for example, the incident report that the LPN on John's floor is required to complete. In actual appearance, the report form is a single sheet of paper with a series of questions relating to its subject's immediate health status and the conditions surrounding an incident. The precise wording of such questions and their format does vary, of course, from one institution to another. In theory, though, regardless of design, reports request information about an *individual*, not principally the subject's social ties or group life. In the case of the bathroom incident, the incident report is expected to contain accurate information about John, *his* condition, and events surrounding *his* accident.

On the report form under consideration, following a question about the patient's or resident's mental condition at the time of the incident is a series of five alternative answers: normal, senile, disoriented, sedated, and other. It is assumed that John cannot logically be both normal and disoriented at the same time; the alternatives are presumed to be mutually exclusive. The LPN responsible for completing the form expects to check one of the five alternatives, not two, three, or more.

The assumption notwithstanding, when Miss Hanson presents the bathroom incident and its consequences to the patient care conference, it is not clear what should be made of John's condition at the time. While the incident report requests that his mental condition be specified according to one of five alternatives, it is evident, too, that in some sense his stumble and the related events of the incident have little to do with whether John, himself, was *actually* normal, disoriented, senile, sedated, or something else. Events relate more to what various parties to the incident *claim* John's condition to be (Spector & Kitsuse, 1977). Miss Hanson implies as much when she says that accepting one alternative over another will be "unfair to someone."

While in theory the contents of the incident report are to be about John, in practice contents are selected from a wide range of other matters. There is the issue of how long the nursing home can continue to accept John as "normal" and keep him on the residential floor. This relates especially to mounting complaints with which the administrator at the time is seriously concerned, by family members about John's presence there. Might it be necessary eventually to consider the possibility that John was actually disoriented or at least not normal enough to be counted as a resident? There also was the question of how the accidents of normal patients or residents in comparison with the accidents of disoriented ones reflect on the facility's quality of care. To a certain extent, it is understandable for a disoriented person to stumble; when normal ones repeatedly have such incidents, it suggests an unsafe environment.

When the associate director of nursing announces, "Welcome to the real world!," one thing is clear: Participants are dealing with events and conditions that are far from straightforward matters of theory. Strictly speaking, to be fair, the incident report might read that John is "senile-for-Phoebe," "normal-for-Sadie," and perhaps "disoriented-for-a-family-member." The hyphenated grammar would signal the reality of perspective. In any event, it is undeniable to Miss Hanson and other participants in the patient care conference that, in the real world—which they all have to contend with—John is many mental statuses at the same time. To dismiss this is unrealistic.

TIES

The real world does not arbitrarily turn problems into troubles. Phoebe did not simply decide all of a sudden that John had "lost his marbles." If problems became troublesome arbitrarily, John's mental status could just as easily have led Phoebe to view John as a conniving genius. In fact, Phoebe does not, and neither do any members of her clique. Their troubles with John have to do with what they feel about him before, during, and after the incident. In the real world, the trouble that a particular problem presents depends on one's relation or *tie* to the person under consideration.

In theory, diseases, needs, dysfunctions, and other problems that professional caregivers are trained to deal with can be diagnosed or assessed, an intervention or treatment designed, an application made, and progress monitored. The entire effort assumes that a problem is discernible and remains stable long enough to treat or otherwise deal with. The professional worker takes for granted that some individual has the problem and that an individual is expected to be cared for. When, less commonly, the object of care or intervention is a group (such as a family), the assumption is, by extension, that the boundaries of the group and its problem are discernible and remain clear long enough to effect intervention.

The interpersonal ties of the real world violate these assumptions and thereby complicate problems. Consider again the bathroom incident, its written report, and events surrounding them. Whether the report explains, or explains away, what actually happened, it nonetheless is meant to be read as being about a series of events that led up to an incident involving an individual whose condition at the time made it likely to occur. If this were all there was to the matter, Miss Hanson and the other staff members who discuss it would have been presented with a straightforward individual matter, namely, John's problem. Staff might have planned to monitor his behavior lest he repeatedly stumble and fall. They might have had John's eyes checked or his needs for daily activity and exercise assessed. Had it been suggested that the reason John heads for any available bathroom or toilet is that he has to urinate frequently, the possibility of incontinence might have been raised.

After the incident and conference, Miss Hanson and others advise John to restrict his walking to shorter distances and more familiar surroundings. Their efforts not only run afoul of John's contrary view of the stumble but his ire at "what *they* are trying to do." While the stumble is called a "fall" by the staff and "just desserts" by Phoebe's clique, the staff soon learns, if they have not already surmised, that John feels otherwise.

In elaborating "what *they* are trying to do," John refers to two different groups of people. In one case, "they" refers to the staff. In complaining to Sadie, John's friend, about what Miss Hanson has advised regarding his perambulations, John remarks that the staff is "really" trying to keep him away from the "old bags." He explains, "I haven't heard anything about them [the staff] telling the old bags to stay away from us." John rails that it is not his stumbling that they are "really" concerned about, but "that goofy Phoebe and her goofy son who complain all the time about everything in here." It is obvious to John that "they," the staff, are trying to make life easy for themselves by keeping him quiet. To John, staff's response to the bathroom incident, the stumble or fall in particular, has nothing to do with his state of mind or caregiving and everything to do with social discrimination.

"They" also refers to those whom John calls "the old bags." John's heated discussions with his friends show that he considers the staff, especially Miss Hanson, to have been manipulated by Phoebe and her clique. It is evident to John that the staff members who have talked to him after the incident are really doing "Phoebe's dirty work." Miss Hanson has not been entirely unaware of this possible interpretation and its repercussions. Following her warning in the patient care conference that whatever the staff does, it will be unfair to someone, Hanson reminds everyone that she really likes John very much and can understand, even sympathize with, how he feels about Phoebe and what John refers to as "those catty women at the other end of the hall." Hanson mentions that she is a bit worried that John might see staff's attempt to help him as taking "their" (the clique's) side. She advises the staff to make it as clear as possible to John that they are concerned about his safety.

Another assumption in theory—the relative stability of a problem—is soon to begin breaking down. After John is counseled about "his" problem, it starts to change markedly, not in degree but in kind. What John has initially denied is a fall, but has admitted is a stumble, soon becomes neither. To John, what happened that morning became clear evidence of staff's attempt to, as he put it, "see whatever I do as wrong." The trouble for John is gradually being transformed into staff's undue attention to Phoebe's claims and staff's resulting inability to approach any goings-on with the proper balance. For staff, Miss Hanson in particular, the trouble is starting to affect the quality of staff-resident relations. This is highlighted on one occasion when John calmly but firmly warns Miss Hanson, "If you all keep keeping an eye on everything that's wrong with me instead of doing something about them old bags down there, things is going to get a lot worse around here."

TRADITIONS

I speak at length with Hanson and other staff members about the incident and its consequences, the place of families in such matters, about troubles, and the related ties of staff and residents. While not everyone is directly involved in the events surrounding the bathroom incident, many have formed opinions about it, part of the continuing flow of gossip and sentiment about daily life in the facility. The talk and judgments reveal that *tradition*, too, contrasts the real world with the ideal. While troubles tell of complications, loose ends, and "things you just can't predict," there also are enduring, interpersonal facts of life to contend with, what people have long meant to each other as well as evolving understandings that take on new momentum of their own.

As time passes, Miss Hanson feels that she might have made matters worse for herself on the residential floor by focusing on John's problem. While he continues to greet her with a smile, their interactions are definitely cool. Before the incident, John had a habit of peeking into Hanson's office after lunch and bantering briefly about the noonday meal. They cherished a harmless joking relationship regarding the quality of food in the home. Each tried to outdo the other in describing how bad it can be. For example, on one occasion, when John scoffs, "It was another day of cardboard and sponges," referring to the texture of the meat and bread served at lunch, Hanson retorts, "Not as bad as my dishwater and linoleum," which evidently more vividly describes her soup and sandwich.

Some time after the bathroom incident, Hanson laments that she now misses John's "drop-ins," wishes the "damn incident hadn't happened," and that she had determined a way to keep "those two" (John and Phoebe) at the opposite ends of the hall. Miss Hanson recalls how she had grown fond of John's daily exchanges with her, brief as they were, and the welcome relief they brought to her workday, "You grow accustomed to them [residents and patients] and their ways and when that changes or they leave, you can miss it." The difficulty is, as another staff member reminds her, "You can't go home again." What had become a ritual post-lunch relationship now has vanished and, it is agreed, cannot easily be restored. Miss Hanson sighs, "I guess there's not much point in asking John to stop by whenever he can, like before, because he'd think I'm trying to counsel him."

Hanson surmises that the trouble she now faces with John might not have become so difficult for her had they not been so fond of each other. While any resident might resent what can be construed as discriminatory intervention, John feels betrayed. The history of their relationship, notably its daily rituals, casts a shadow of its own on an existing tie and the emergent interpersonal meaning of trouble.

That the real world appears to have a greater share of undesirable than desirable traditions is all too evident in "bitch sessions," where the real world is described as full of entrenched ways of doing things and unbending attitudes. The residential floor of this nursing home is said to have many undesirable traditions, like the habit of hostility between John's and Phoebe's group. The tradition makes the respective troubles of residential ties worse than they otherwise might have been. The tradition has its ritual underpinnings, carried out in what staff believe to be a totally irrational manner. Nothing seems to precipitate its rhythms except tradition itself. It has become a custom for John to "hiss" Phoebe and other members of her clique, just as it has become a habit for Phoebe to loudly but seemingly inadvertently disparage John and his friends in public. When staff attempt to account for this and other rituals, a typical explanation is that things have always been that way and will undoubtedly continue.

There are traditions in family relations too. Following any untoward incident on the first floor, Miss Hanson can expect a ritual complaint from Phoebe's son. She realizes that she cannot dismiss her own ritual response to it. As the administrator once remarked about complaints in sympathy with his staff, "You have to learn to dance with these cat-and-mouse games most of the time or they'll eat you alive." Staff responses to the real world of frail elderly and their families, like families' responses, can be equally set. As custom varies, so does the meaning of troubles and the ties that drive them.

The Mosaic of Care

In an article on the experience of daughters caring for elderly mothers, Lewis and Meredith (1988) distinguish two ways of viewing caregiving relationships. One is the common approach of professional workers who see caregiving in what the authors call "linear" terms, figuring needs on the basis of the professional's own skills and discipline rather than from the subjectively meaningful, multifaceted ties and traditions of those involved in caregiving. Lewis and Meredith point out that the approach "may therefore tend either to displace [the family or nonprofessional] carer rather than supplement her work, or to offer help which the carer or person cared for perceives as inappropriate to their needs" (p. 9). Citing Waerness (1984), the authors add that the approach combines with the increasing fragmentation of human service to pick apart the primary caregiving relationship, not give it the total attention it deserves. Linear, or service-oriented, models overshadow what Lewis and Meredith describe as the "reality of the complex set of caring relationships."

Lewis and Meredith's own view reflects an alternate approach, oriented to the real world of frail elderly and their relations with families. Citing Evers (1983, 1985), the authors write that studying the caregiver alone is insufficient and that a focus on the complex relationship is paramount. Referring to the importance of taking interpersonal traditions into account, they indicate that proper understanding must steer clear of a "snapshot" approach and include a view of the history of the relationship as well as its extended social ties. Lewis and Meredith refer to this broader context as a "caring matrix."

DISTINGUISHING MOSAIC FROM CONTINUUM

The distinction between the linear view and the view toward a caring matrix is a basis for distinguishing the overall *mosaic of care* from what commonly is called a "continuum" of care. A continuum of care is a service-oriented spectrum of administrative caregiving options. The mosaic of care emphasizes caring's distinct and complex interpersonal experiences.

Linearity versus complexity. Continuum implies length and order, suggesting that the experience of caring can be aligned in some way. A common alignment is in terms of the professional skills required to care for those in need. At one end of the continuum is care requiring few professional skills and little intervention; at the other end is care provided by the most skilled professionals.

This may be expressed as a spectrum of care organizations. For example, in classifying what they call "old-age institutions," Manard, Kart, and Gils (1975) place extended care and skilled nursing facilities at one end of their continuum of care, and board-and-care or "rest" homes at the other end. Other care organizations, such as chronic disease hospitals and homes for the mentally and physically handicapped, fall at the more skilled end. Since these authors concentrate on formal organizations, the caring household does not figure in the continuum. McPherson (1983) presents a more complex schema, combining the criteria of dependency and segregation. At one end of an implicit continuum, labeled "housing alternatives for the elderly" (p. 298), are options based on age segregation and dependency, such as nursing homes and long-term care and psychiatric hospitals. At the other end are housing alternatives combining age integration and independence, such as homes, apartments, and single-room occupancy hotels. While a continuum of care for frail elderly is drawn from McPherson's two-dimensional scheme, it is more broadly a classification of living arrangements for the elderly as a whole.

What is defined in theory as according with particular professional skills does not necessarily translate into practice. Commenting on this issue in relation to what she generally calls "supportive housing," Hilker (1987) states that select settings at one end of the continuum of supportive housing may be just as "home-like" as at the other end. What is more, particular facilities at one end may offer as many or varied services as facilities at the other end. Citing a study by the American Bar Association (1983), Hilker adds that since licensing standards tend to center on food services, staffing ratios, the physical plant, and administrative regulations, there is no guarantee, in practice, that "residents and services [will be] appropriately matched or [that] there is actual delivery of services after placement" (p. 239). Linearity may actually hide more complex care environments.

Continuity versus discontinuity. A continuum of care also implies continuity, that is, a continuous gradation of differences in needs and services. Yet, while the skilled nursing home or chronic care hospital may be placed at the high end of the continuum of care, and the caring household at the other end, there can be gaps in between. As Hilker's term "supportive housing" suggests, between the extremes are such contexts of caring as adult daycare, shared housing, board-and-care homes, adult congregate living facilities, personal care or residential units of nursing homes, and possibly the life care facilities that combine both ends of the continuum in one setting.

The professional worker who orients to the length and continuity of a continuum of care envisions caregiving options in terms of what Lewis and Meredith call a linear, or service-oriented, view. For example, while a case manager who finds a frail elderly person growing weak and helpless may attempt to keep the elder at home or in the community as long as possible, in a broad linear orientation, the case manager plans for options farther down the continuum of care as possible future placements. The linear orientation attunes the case manager to a service-oriented panorama of care, not the complex matrix of care defined by the care receiver, significant others, and family members, which may be anything but linearly aligned or continuous in its understanding of alternatives.

This does not mean that the personal sentiments of professional workers do not come into play, like the individual case manager who prefers community placements for frail elderly regardless of the direction of flow in theory of an ostensible continuum of care. But individual exceptions may be set against human service systems guided by different professional principles, articulating intervention according to the widely held spectrum of options, one with a linear and continuous patterning.

Rational planning versus understanding. The linearity and continuity built into the idea of a continuum of care provide for rational, administratively defined planning. In relation to the real world, however, planning encounters the caring matrix, that is, the complex and emergent definitions of care receivers and their families, as well as administrative perspectives. Because in the real world these definitions present diverse troubles to be dealt with as much as problems to be cared for, a different sense of intervention is indicated, oriented to the dynamic interplay of troubles, ties, and traditions. The professional caregiver needs to *understand*, not predefine, the meaning of problems. Preferably, he or she aims to facilitate the inventive recovery of troubled lives, not preplan for them. The very concept of rational planning works against this understanding of recovery.

STORY AND VERSION

The alternate sense of intervention requires a suitable language. I began to form such a language by describing the troubles, ties, and interpersonal traditions of frail elderly, families, professional workers, and their network of social relations. Lewis and Meredith's term "caring matrix" adds a handy challenge to the continuum of care, focusing as it does on ties and traditions beyond the formal service relationship.

Though useful, the idea of a caring matrix is not broad enough. The real world is a configuration of interpretations as much as it is an array of problems, cares, and interpersonal linkages. Thus I add *story* to the language of troubles, ties, and traditions. A proper tolerance and respect for emergent meanings and storied patternings as well as the interactional complexities Meredith and Lewis highlight provide a basis for intervention respectful of subjectively meaningful experiences, a mosaic indeed.

Return to the nursing home incident in this broader context. As far as the completion of an incident report for John's "accident" was concerned, John had a concrete problem. He had fallen or stumbled and hurt himself, his mental status perhaps causing the accident. In practice, the problem could not easily be disentangled from the troubles it presented from various perspectives. The problem in theory was a variety of troubles in practice. Troubles were not simply arbitrary definitions, but were related to social ties and traditions.

This real world was as much a configuration of interpretations—stories—differentially told by those concerned as it was a matrix of concrete events and relationships. Yes, something had happened in the bathroom. Those at the actual scene of events, John and Lillian, had either observed with their own eyes or heard with their own ears that a man and a woman were occupying the room simultaneously, something they knew in principle to be undesirable, if not outrageous. Yet what was seen or heard by John, Lillian, and others had strikingly different meanings.

All concerned responded to the fuss over what happened; what actually happened could not be separated from perspective. Take Miss Hanson for instance. While she knew that something had occurred in the bathroom at the clique's end of the hallway, she was frustrated that it came in so many *versions*. Miss Hanson heard one story from Phoebe and another from John. The LPN on the floor conveyed yet another. Later, as Hanson tried to sort things out, still other versions presented themselves. Each was either directly told by someone or was derived from testimony and behaviors. Knowing who told a story seemed to throw as much light on events as the events themselves.

In response to a family complaint, the administrator suggested Miss Hanson look into the matter immediately. Her actions in investigating the incident created stories of their own. For example, John conveyed a story of things to come, warning Miss Hanson that a persistent negative appraisal of his conduct would just make matters worse. While, in theory, stories are meant to represent events in the real world, Miss Hanson's experience showed that stories were an actual part of it.

When Miss Hanson and I discussed the bathroom incident a few weeks later, she told me that she had done all she could about it. Things had not changed much between John, Phoebe, and their respective circles of friends, even though her relations with John had. Hanson remarked that, "people being what they are," she expected more of the same any day now, but was not sure exactly when. She added that nonetheless, as before, she would try to do what she could to intervene effectively, no matter what happened. Her remarks indicated that troubles, ties, and traditions were continually productive of stories. The comment, "people being what they are" suggested as much.

The remarks were a story in their own right—a story about stories—about what Phoebe, John, and others, including Miss Hanson herself, had said concerning the bathroom incident. The stories not only diversely articulated the real world but they reconstructed it. As Hanson once tellingly chided indirectly referring to my field-work in the nursing home, "You might get a different story from me next month."

Just as John, Phoebe, Miss Hanson, and others had their stories, they also conveyed stories about each other's stories. While what Phoebe had told Hanson about John was important to Miss

Hanson, of equal significance to Hanson was what John had conveyed to her about what he believed Phoebe had told Hanson. Also important, yet exasperating, to Hanson was that she was obliged to interpret coherently, and respond to fairly, what she had been told by all parties. Indeed, when Hanson once thought on the matter at my behest, she stated that "maybe what you have to do in the end is just say what you have to, to whoever." The statement suggested that stories themselves, like the real world that both contains and generates them, are necessarily varied, disjointed, emergent, and inconclusive because stories are both about ties, troubles, and traditions and produced by them—a dynamic mosaic.

Story, Theme, and Local Culture

Just as novels are part of a world of literature, not just produced out of individual authors' experiences, ordinary stories of everyday life are not private narratives but are informed by shared understandings. Phoebe's, John's, Miss Hanson's, and others' stories take on their meaning in relation to the varied life *themes* typifying experience in a place like a nursing home, themes such as confusion, loss of home, abandonment, adjustment, and dementia. This does not mean that individual stories are mere copies of what is shared, only that stories pick up on the typical concerns and experiential categories of a setting. The common life themes of a setting are part of its *local culture* (Gubrium, 1989a), a term adapted from anthropologists who use culture to refer to the more or less contained meanings and categories shared by a group of people (Geertz, 1983). Local culture is a more organizationally delimited version of culture, stressing place and circumstance. Theme and local culture add further to the language of the mosaic of care.

DISTINGUISHING THEME AND PLOT

Each story heard about residents in the facility where Miss Hanson worked contains something typical of nursing home cultures as well as particular matters—theme and plot respectively. Phoebe's complaint about John's behavior and his mental status thematizes a common experiential concern in a setting like a nursing home, expressed in hallmark categories like *"non compos mentis"* and "lost marbles." The precise events recounted in Phoebe's story plot the occurrences that vex her and her circle of friends.

The distinction between theme and plot is commonly, if perhaps tacitly, recognized. Miss Hanson, a nurse, and I once struck up a conversation about residents who were said to talk to themselves. The nurse commented that she was a bit worried that a resident, Nancy, might not be suited to residential living. Apparently, Nancy's roommate, Betty, had mentioned several times that Nancy talked to herself and could not find their room. The talking and confusion disturbed Betty because it made her think that she herself might one day "lose her mind." Without using the word "theme," the nurse added that this was, "of course, the typical kind of stuff you hear all the time."

Recounting the *kinds* of stories one regularly hears in a nursing home, Hanson and the nurse spoke in general about what was being shared. At one point, Miss Hanson turned to me and asked if I had not, by now, heard the same stories. (At the time, I'd been doing fieldwork in the home for several months.) When I responded that I had, many times, the nurse asserted, "Yeah and if you've heard them once, you've heard them all." She explained that she had worked in several nursing homes, heard many stories and complaints, and that, except for details, had yet to hear anything that was "that different" from what was being presently considered.

I was particularly interested in references to kinds of stories because they suggested themes were being distinguished from individual plots or story lines. While stories of John's intimate overtures had led to complaints of his possible mental incompetence, which of course differed in detail from stories and complaints (or "concerns") conveyed about Nancy's confusion, they were, nonetheless, a kind of story allegedly common to nursing home life. The stories were familiar because their broad outlines reflected themes that staff members regularly referenced and took into account.

Theme was signaled in several ways. The most common was to speak of a "kind" of story. Less common were references to "the same old story," "familiar stories," and "the same old song and dance," among other expressions. When I explicitly used theme and plot myself in the manner under consideration, the difference was immediately recognized. For example, when I remarked that certain stories I had heard had a familiar theme, responses suggested that it was not plot so much as it was a kind of story—a theme—that was focal.

Yet all knew, too, that stories were more than themes. When I mentioned a particular theme or a kind of story I had been accustomed to hearing, I was likely to be asked about whom I was talking, what I had in mind, or another question focused on particulars. In this way, local culture was always subject to specification and embellishment, the typical continually being articulated by the particular.

EXEMPLARS AS THEMES

Some stories virtually stood for a theme, their subjects being exemplars. While John's conduct, for one, was not considered by all to thematize mental demise, his story could nonetheless be compared to exemplars of what could happen to anyone's faculties in later life whose behavior and circumstances resembled John's.

On one occasion, a group of residents had gathered in the day lounge and were discussing various personalities. John was not present. John's friend, Sadie, commented that she thought John had cooled down in the last few weeks but that he might have been a bit shaken by his stumble and all the trouble it had caused. While Sadie did not condemn John's actions, she expressed concern for his well-being, especially as it might be affected by events surrounding the bathroom incident and John's continuing poor relations with Phoebe's clique. Sadie noted that it was "probably pretty hard on the fellow to always have a bunch of women like them on his back." Another resident, Melba, joked that her husband used to say that too many old women around would get any man down. This caused considerable laughter and scoffing.

Melba extended the discussion of John's mood of late, commenting that she had seen "it happen a lot." She pointed out that what often happens when someone (older) has an accident like a fall or an operation is that "it" can lead to forgetfulness and "all the rest." Mike, another resident, immediately chimed in, "Yeah, like what happened to George," continuing:

> Remember when he [George] fell and broke his hip? [Several confirmed that they remembered very well.] Before that he was all piss and vinegar. But when he came back from the hospital, he just wasn't the same at all. That guy took a tumble, just like John, and he lost his

marbles right after that. There was just no way he could have his old room back. Remember how they tried him out down the hall for a while, but he really never did know where he was and what was going on after that. They didn't have much choice, did they? I wonder how he's getting along upstairs?

The group recounted George's resistance to being transferred to an intermediate care floor, sympathizing with George, yet acknowledging that he was no longer fit to remain among them. Whether or not there is any factual link between bodily accidents and mental demise in old age, the group believed that a link explained what happened to George. Indeed, when Mike later stated and others acknowledged that "it could happen to any one of us," it was evident that George's story exemplified a theme that could underscore any of their stories.

Mike warned that John better be careful because "it" (John's fall and its alleged possible impact on his mental state) could have been a lot worse. Sadie responded that she knew what Mike meant, but that John was no George, explaining that John had more wits about him than George ever did. Another member of the group was more skeptical and warned that if he were John, he'd still be careful because "all that jumping around and cussedness can get you in the end." Even exceptions could exemplify themes.

SETTINGS AS THEMES

Setting and place, too, were thematized. Many stories compared institutional living with home life. The meaning of home was a constant theme in decisions surrounding admission, transfers between levels of care, and discharge. While Phoebe, John, Sadie, and others resided on the premises of a nursing home, they were not patients. Only those on other floors, in need of intermediate or skilled nursing care, were patients. At the same time, the stories the residents shared about such matters as falls, stumbles, and confusion, on the one hand, and hospitalization, institutionalization, and other placements, on the other, reminded them that the setting was an important source of meaning in their immediate lives—a concrete indicator of who they were (residents) and what they might become (patients).

Other settings and places signaled different themes. The household as a source of home care, for example, was thematized in stories of warm family life and tender loving care. Even while some households were depicted as anything but kind and giving, their negative character derived its meaning from a shared positive image of hearth and home. Like other nursing facilities, even the nursing home in which John lived borrowed from this and emulated themes of domesticity in public messages about the provision of a home-like atmosphere.

The Real World and Linear Thinking

While the professional worker is trained in skills to intervene effectively in people's lives, the lives have diverse social orders of their own. What it means for an elderly person to be forgetful on the residential floor of a nursing home in the context of its local culture may be one more indication of someone's growing dementia. What it means in the context of the household of a family that has normalized the bodily and cognitive frailties of late life is quite the opposite—one more sign of aging. Where the one setting categorizes disease, the other circumstance designates normal aging. Of course, not every household normalizes the frailties of aging. Indeed, the growing public culture of the Alzheimer's disease movement may soon convince all that, as the popular exhortation goes, "Alzheimer's disease is *not* normal aging!" (Gubrium, 1986a). Nor is all residential living for elderly linked as closely to nursing care as the unit and floor housing John, Phoebe, and others.

The separate experiences and contexts of the real world resist linear thinking. As Miss Hanson once taught in distinguishing theory from practice, "every social worker worth her salt knows that in the real world you have to take every situation on its own terms," cautioning "no two are exactly alike." Thus the real world's mosaic is taken into account, ranging over troubles, ties, traditions, story, theme, and local culture.

CHAPTER 2

Frail Elderly in the Community

In contrast to family caregivers, who usually work in the home, the activities of professional service providers are typically sponsored by formal organizations. Settings such as the rehabilitation center, nursing home, clinic, hospital, and adult congregate living facility locate much of their work with frail elderly. Even day and respite care are likely to be attached in some way to formal organizations.

For better or worse, organizational categories and contingencies serve as the framework for providing service. While the nurse's aide, for one, is charged with "bed-and-body work"—attending to the cleanliness of patients' bodies and the orderliness of their immediate environs—caregiving is circumscribed by the aide's job description and prevailing work conditions. What passes for care is not just a matter of good or bad intentions or the level of service but accords with organizational practice. In this regard, the elderly are as much official objects as they are persons with individual needs and desires.

Those who work in formal care organizations distinguish elderly served in those settings from elderly in the so-called community. They speculate on, or attempt to assess, what will happen to the older person who returns to the community. They compare what the lives of elderly served were like in the community before they entered the formal care setting. In the process, references to *the* community are heard, as if it were a homogeneous domain, wholly comparable with the care receiver's contrasting experience in the organizational setting. There is a sense in which the sum and substance of this idea of the community is an organizationally produced fiction, a useful source of contrasts for what is done for frail elderly in the formal care setting. As far as the provision of care is concerned, the care setting offers what the community does not.

Take the discharge planning of a treatment team in a rehabilitation hospital (Gubrium & Buckholdt, 1982). The team is composed of the patient's social worker, a nurse, and the patient's physical and occupational therapists. In planning for discharge, prospects for suitable housing are taken into account. Questions of safety, need fulfillment, and custody are considered. Will the patient's own, unoccupied home now be safe enough for one whose speech and communication has been impaired? Does the patient's paralysis make it necessary for him or her to be supervised? How does the patient's personality figure into prospects for adjustment following discharge? Is this the type of person who will readily accept supervision or being housed with others?

While the community presents several options for placement, it nonetheless is what the hospital is not. It is not a treatment setting. For the most part, it is not girded by professionals. It is not rationalized into treatment schedules so that a patient lacking self-monitoring skills is kept on target by the sheer force of institutional schedules such as the written daily treatment regimen or the timing of medication orders. A simple glance at the daily schedule located in the physical therapy gym indicates when the patient is to be in hydrotherapy, when in occupational therapy, when in his or her own room, and so on. It also lists the service responsible for completing a treatment. Indeed, the hospital hires "runners" whose job is to make sure patients are in the right place at the right time; runners take patients to various services and return them to their rooms afterward. In the process of bringing together a virtual armory of efforts to keep the patient "on schedule," the patient's needs and safety are monitored and managed. By and large, the community does not provide this rationalized system of support and care.

Serious and urgent concern over what will happen to the patient when he or she returns to the community tends to homogenize lives. While discharge planners and other professional caregivers engage in community assessments, the basic categories of assessment are distinguished according to a contrast defined in terms of the availability in the community of services the organization provides.

Community Stations and Multiple Realities

Consider Frankfather's (1977) informative study of community responses to senility and deviance as a point of departure for showing how diverse in practice are the troubles, ties, and traditions of frail elderly in community settings. Rather than examining service-defined difficulties of the aged in the community, Frankfather raises a prior question that dehomogenizes community: What can be discerned about the lives of the frail elderly, the "senile" in particular, if community is treated as a varied field of contacts with service agents, organizations, and interested others, each presenting separate understandings of problems?

As Frankfather sees it, the community does not present itself wholesale to frail elderly, but as "stations" with distinctly targeted missions. The term is meant to indicate that there are community stopping points at which elderly encounter persons or agents concerned for their well-being or whereabouts. Among the specific community stations considered are the family, the nursing home, the senior citizen center, the "Main Street luncheonette," and the geriatric outreach agency. The mentally impaired aged who come into contact with the ideology or interpretive categories of one station do not necessarily encounter the same understanding of their conduct and condition as they do at another station. The accountings of the different stations show each problem to be multiple realities, diverse troubles according to the varied viewpoints of station agents.

Frankfather conducts participant observation in a community named "Claiborne," which is a distinct section of a large metropolitan area. Claiborne is mostly white, approximately 16 percent of its 44,000 residents being elderly. It is predominantly low-income with a sprinkling of wealthy homes. Some large houses have been converted into residential care facilities. There are health, mental health, and social services located nearby.

Frankfather distinguishes two principle responses to elderly in the community: the preservation of social order disrupted by troubled individuals and the rehabilitation of the troubled individual. Different Claiborne stations and agents stress one principle or the other, some attempting to control the senile aged's troublemaking to keep the peace and others seeking to treat the source of the troublemaking. The strategy of the mental hospital is to stabilize the troubles produced by mental impairment. In contrast, the strategy of the police is to restore the order that troubles disrupt, say, by transporting a confused, combative elderly person out of the community.

The ideologies of treatment and control affect community responses to the aged in different ways. Being control-oriented, the police attempt to eliminate the public nuisance of the troublemaker, considering their job done when the troublesome have been sequestered. Treatment-oriented stations or agents begin their work at the point a troubled individual is secured. Altogether, the orientations represent quite diverse, some might say contradictory, community commitments. From the point of view of the impaired elderly, encounters with community members are quite disjointed, ranging from containment to challenges to self-definition. Against the background of diverse purposes, one can hardly simply speak of elderly in *the* community.

The diversity is magnified when acquaintance and friendship ties are taken into account. While the police and treatment agents respond to the troubles of mental impairment in different ways, they nonetheless regularly use the language of senility or dementia to frame their respective concerns. Nonprofessional friends and acquaintances of the mentally impaired, however, are less likely to refer to troubles in terms of pathology. Frankfather notes that while some of the mentally impaired are considered dangerous, others are believed to be a minor nuisance. As three customers at a community luncheonette explain:

> There's nothing else for them to do but bum cigarettes. It's a kind of social exchange.

> I gave him a quarter and said, "Now don't tell or they'll all be after me."

> There's one mean one. If you don't give him cigarettes, he'll ask for money. He steals candy from little children. Or he waits for them to come out of the candy store and takes their change (pp. 28–29).

As two firefighters observe about the confused elderly in commenting on passersby:

> *Most of them are just lonely. They'll talk to you all day if you let them. I try to avoid them.*
>
> *They like to talk to people in uniform. It gives them a sense of recognition. It makes them feel good (p. 29).*

In presenting testimony from an elderly panhandler, Frankfather explains that what is confused and pathological to some can be seen as legitimate economic pursuit by others. As one ostensibly confused panhandler remarks:

> *I only got one dollar a week from the nursing home. They wouldn't even give me money for a haircut. I make about two dollars a day. It used to be better but a police detective caught me and said if he saw me doing it again, he'd throw me in the clinker. So now I just go up and down the side streets (p. 29).*

We come away from Frankfather's book with the sense that, in the real world, community is a set of diverse contrasts and, according to its separate narrators, a place of multiple realities and stories. In tracing varied accounts of confused elderly in the community, Frankfather describes lives virtually oscillating between distinct troubles. Contrasting themes such as pathology, social control, and daily travail make dubious the applicability of a linear continuum of experiences.

Community Types

There is a way in which professional workers in organized care settings informally diversify, by classifying frail elderly into community types, what they otherwise treat as uniform. Staff members reference typical instances of, say, how patient *A* versus patient *B* is likely to respond to a particular placement. In estimating how patient *A* will fare when she returns to the community, staff specify that this type of person or placement makes for a quick, easy, or difficult adjustment, according to the type indicated. Answers to the community care questions raised earlier are constructed out of estimates of the type of person a particular patient is believed to be. In the process, professional workers bridge the gap between the homogeneous community on the one side and the many and diverse patients with whom they come into contact on the other. The use of types tells how lives known in considerable detail (the elderly patient) will respond in a domain that is relatively uncontrolled and undistinguished.

The word "type" actually is used in the process of deliberation. For example, it might be said that patient X is a fiercely independent type and he or she is likely to require few community support services. Types are also contrasted. A fiercely independent type, for instance, contrasts with the homebody, who is said to need the constant cocoon of domestic security to survive in the community. Sometimes, even "classic" types are indicated, such as the classic familial dependent who "just can't seem to make it on [his or her] own." The shared recognition of types, in particular classic types, is validated in statements like "you [we] know the type."

There may be disagreement about the type an individual patient or client represents. For some, a particular patient may be a fiercely independent type and thus not justify detailed discharge planning. For others, the same patient may be said to "actually" be an entirely different type for which careful monitoring is required.

Types are subject to specification. The concrete characteristics of a type are assigned to characteristics of the individual to whom the label is applied. When an elderly patient, Ben, whose story will be presented shortly, is labeled fiercely independent or simply an independent type, the specification of the type Ben is, in turn, is concretely exemplified by Ben's own character and conduct. As such, each type is tailored to individual particulars on the one hand, while taken to be a general engagement with the community on the other.

The particulars of types come in the form of more or less detailed stories. For example, the question of how patient X is likely to do in the community because she is a particular type is compared and contrasted with discharged patient Y's community experience, who it is said is the same or another type. Patient Y's story provides a basis for decision making concerning patient X's discharge and placement. Stories mediate the unknowns of what actually happens to elders in the community with what is known and believed about elderly in the context of the formal care setting.

Consider four prominent community types and exemplary stories conveyed by professional workers. While the types are general and the individuals particular, they combine in practice. Each story has related themes. Story lines are complicated by the attributed troubles, circumscribing ties, and existing traditions of their characters. Family figures significantly in the stories because troubles commonly link the home or homelessness with professional service provision.

The Fiercely Independent: Ben's Story

Ben's story of fierce independence is anyone's of his type. While certain details differentiate the plot of his story from others, what is conveyed in its broad outline as a kind of community existence is much the same. There are many Ben-like stories, about any man or woman in ostensible need whose life, it is said, defies every effort to intervene effectively.

I heard Ben's story from a case manager who worked for a small United Fund elderly care project in a large, Midwestern industrial city (Gubrium, 1973). As Dorothy, the case manager, tells it, Ben is one of "those types" from whom "you just can't get anything straight." Dorothy states that it is virtually impossible to complete a fact sheet for Ben, that is, the summary background information one usually first finds in a case file. Dorothy explains that for Ben's type, one never knows very much because "they" always seem to be hiding details of their lives from you. Indeed, after countless visits to Ben's hotel, she does not know for sure if he has any living relatives or local friends.

Ben lives alone in a single-room occupancy, or SRO, hotel. Always either too hot or too cold, it is located on a busy thoroughfare. His room is full of grime and dust from the street, and is, according to Dorothy, the kind of housing that "you can immediately see shows he is having real problems getting by." Ben has no telephone and is not easy to reach. She tries many times to find him at the hotel to no avail. When she leaves messages for him at what appears to be the front desk, they are never delivered or answered. To Dorothy, Ben is an urban nomad; he has a place, yes, but it seems to be more an oasis where he might or might not be found, depending on his seemingly incomprehensible daily schedule.

When Dorothy does find him in his room or on the street, he keeps his distance, indulging her concern only to the extent she can do something for him. For Ben she is part of an agenda for survival that has no place in it for what Dorothy needs to do as part of her job, such as securing information on the client, organizing a service strategy, seeing to the client's needs, and monitoring his whereabouts.

The worst of it is that the few details Dorothy has come to accept—his name, address, age, lack of family—are murky. For example, she believes his name is Ben Beale; at least that's what she usually calls him and what he initially responded to. She has that on record. But this is not what she hears at the nearby diner. There he is called "Bud," "BB," "Stan," or "Mike." When she addresses him by any of these names, he reacts with suspicion. In fact, his confusion at one point suggests that Ben might be mentally impaired. In time, though, Dorothy dismisses that possibility as Ben inadvertently comments that one has to have several aliases "on the street" because there are so many different things, people, friends, enemies, and unknowns that one has to deal with, day in and day out. Dorothy surmises that in a world like Ben's, a name can be a handicap because it assigns too much identity to a life that needs to be flexible enough to be known in many ways in order to get by or to keep from being easily located. Dorothy learns that what Ben can't get, maybe "Stan" can or that what "Stan" owes, "BB" perhaps does not.

Dorothy is troubled by Ben's transience. He has a room, of course, but she hears from others whom she speaks with at the hotel or in the immediate vicinity that he "lives" at a variety of other places. Ben seems to resent the fact that Dorothy knows some of their locations. He prefers his infrequent contact with Dorothy to be at her store-front office, not on his varied turfs.

The case not only is difficult but notably anti-interventionist. After we become acquainted, Dorothy mentions several times, "You know the type." What she means is that Ben doesn't want help; he wants, as Dorothy puts it, "only what *he* wants and on his own terms." Ben sees the limited world he has access to as a platter of options and offerings, meager as they are. He does not frame what he picks and chooses in terms of help, never taking himself to be a client in the conventional sense of the word. Dorothy explains that from Ben's point of view what becomes available to him, through professional service intervention or otherwise, are simply goods. To call what he wants or lacks "needs" and the things offered to him "services" are far from the meaning they are assigned by Ben. At times, Dorothy sighs that the real world seems to be full of Bens, that is, filled with those who resist being categorized in terms she is obliged to deal with.

Ben's story is unusual only in that he carries to an extreme what Dorothy believes to be the fiercely independent grip on life. It is defined as much in opposition to the relatively rationalized and fixed features of service intervention as by the sovereignty of such lives in their own right.

Dorothy thinks Ben is about 70 years old. He mentions a number of ages. There are hints that Ben might have family ties of some kind in the city, perhaps a son. Then again, Ben sometimes swears he has no family, has never married, and could not have supported a family in any case. Dorothy cannot get a handle on any social attachments. As Dorothy tells Ben's story, she says it is typical of the fiercely independent that they seem to survive on their own. Still, it seems typical, too, that there might be ties that refuse to be identified for one reason or another, the reasons themselves typically being equally unclear.

Ben refrains from accommodating Dorothy's sense of his troubles. She does what she can for Ben; his sporadic gratitude suggests that she is fulfilling some need. For example, while he refuses to take advantage of a scheduled optometric examination, he nonetheless thanks her for giving him enough money to buy a pair of cheap, over-the-counter glasses and pocket the difference. Whenever she feels successful in alleviating one of Ben's problems, his appreciation serves to redefine what is accomplished from intervention to gratuitous exchange. His troubles continually work at cross-purposes with her own.

As Dorothy tells it, Ben's world has a dynamic of its own. While Dorothy does not use the term "tradition," she conveys Ben's life over the long haul as rent with constant fits, starts, and lately with loose ends for her. As far as Dorothy can tell, it is a life full of concertedly self-defined troubles and nebulous ties. The tradition of loose ties and ends make intervention anything but easy.

Like other stories, Ben's tells of a type that diversifies what is "out there." Its sharing gives shape and substance to what otherwise is a homogeneous community.

"The Unexpected Community": Rita's Story

Some years ago, sociologist Arlie Hochschild (1973) took advantage of a job as assistant recreation director in a small, low-income apartment building for elderly near San Francisco Bay to study patterns of social integration. What she observed at Merrill Court, the housing project studied, was an unexpected community of grandmothers. She had expected to find 43 isolated and lonely people. Instead, Hochschild discovered an intricately woven network of sentiments and attachments.

There are many stories about life in such settings, where elderly live in close proximity, housed under a common roof but maintain separate homes (apartments). The housing may be set aside for the elderly at considerable discount and offer recreational programs and support services such as transportation to supermarkets and churches, limited onsite medical screenings, and monthly clinics.

Rita's story, like Hochschild's account of life at Merrill Court, tells of the unexpected. Rita lives in Burton Place, a high-rise, low-income apartment building in a working class neighborhood, the kind of public housing for elderly found in many cities (Gubrium, 1973). Her story conveys local troubles, ties, and traditions that are not formally organized but seem to grow out of the daily contacts and concerns of life on such premises. Where the troubles posed by a life like Ben's present fierce independence and an anti-service tenor, Rita's story reveals a "hidden" configuration of interdependencies that can precipitously complicate the meaning of human needs, resources, support, and intervention.

A visiting nurse, Anne, conveys Rita's story to me and others. Working out of the local health department, Anne makes weekly and sometimes daily visits to the varied public housing sites in the vicinity. She provides health and educational services such as monitoring blood pressures and conducting regular personal care classes for residents and interested outsiders. Burton's residents look forward to her visits and confide in her.

Rita is a relatively long-time resident of Burton Place. She moved into the building when she was 72 years old and now is 76. Before that, she lived alone in what her daughter thought was "too much house" for a frail, widowed, elderly woman. It was a three-bedroom bungalow located in an old style ethnic neighborhood not too far from a major automobile plant. The plant had provided Rita's husband a job for the greater part of his life. When all her children had left home and, later when Rita's husband died, she became one more widow residing in a neighborhood that was slowly changing its character, housing younger families without the ethnicity Rita and others had known.

Rita had been both pleased and apprehensive about the move to Burton. She was pleased to have the opportunity to be in a place with people like herself, mostly widowed and from a similar background. But she had felt that Burton would lack the familiar surroundings of her own home and, because it was an apartment building, would mean she would forever be in the company of strangers. She found out differently.

Describing life in "places like Burton," Anne presents richly detailed connections and meanings. Few residents lack local ties. When Anne refers to the one or two loners among them, she makes it clear that the status "loner" is uncommon and to be rectified, not to be accepted. Anne explains that it is very difficult to maintain a solitary lifestyle at Burton because, for better or worse, everyone is either looking out for the other, sharing the latest gossip, or "at each other's throats."

Similar to what Hochschild finds at Merrill Court, Rita's story reflects a local culture of institutionalized thoughtfulness. Participants take it upon themselves to make sure no resident is forgotten on holidays, anniversaries, or other special occasions. Everyone receives small gifts at Christmas and is sent cards on birthdays, at Easter, and on Valentine's Day. What had been an apprehensive move to Burton for Rita is a life replete with social ties, filled with belonging.

Anne explains that because life in such places is so full and interesting, it can be difficult for a service provider. The difficulty for Anne centers on a life theme quite at odds with themes Ben's type presents. Dorothy has difficulty keeping track of Ben and organizing interventions because he resents dependence of any kind. Rita's story, in contrast, is a tale of mutual support, interdependence, and social obligation. Anne has to be very careful what she tells the residents, for their mutual obligation to share information about each other, especially health-related, makes rumors fly.

The residents generally believe that any health problem one resident experiences is likely to be a difficulty another one will experience. Newly contracted, individual health problems are an omen for all residents to take appropriate precautions, which means that there is a need to "tell all" at the slightest hint of ill health, as Anne explains.

One time, in connection with the sharing of health news, Anne finds to her dismay that an individual consultation with Rita about her diet eventually mushrooms into a local food panic and dietary distress. Rita mentions to Anne that she has consulted her doctor because of recent constipation. Her doctor has recommended that she get more exercise and alter her diet. When Anne offers suggestions of her own about particular foods that might help, she inadvertently states in jest, "They're even saying that food sometimes can prevent certain forms of cancer." Immediately after Anne makes the comment, she wonders whether she should have said anything at all. The suggestion develops into collective distress among residents. As Anne suspected, Rita soon tells her next-door neighbor, who in turn probably informs her friend on the next floor, who then speaks to her neighbor, and so on. From the many residents who quickly and anxiously come to Anne either for nutrition advice or for more information about which foods "cause" cancer, Anne knows that trouble lies ahead.

What was originally an innocent comment to Rita about food and cancer prevention grows into a series of accusations by family members and the resident manager that Anne is scaring everyone by giving them poor health advice. Making matters worse is that Rita has become one of three central figures in the residential gossip network. According to Anne, anything Rita says spreads like wildfire. Rita is highly respected. Whatever she conveys not only is quickly consumed, but touted too. It is just Anne's bad luck to have made the inadvertent comment to Burton's "human microphone," as Anne puts it.

There is, of course, another side to Rita's story. Anne describes the warm and kindly person she otherwise finds Rita to be—the traditional helping hand who always is available when there is a project to complete. In this regard, Rita's type, for Anne, accords with a theme of residential life at large—social integration. Still, these very social facts and theme can be a source of trouble for the professional worker. In this circumstance, with its particular ties and traditions, intervention that inadvertently assumes residents to be individuals is shortsighted. As Anne explains, "At Burton, when you deal with one, you can be sure you're dealing with them all." As if to underscore Rita's story line in this regard, Anne concludes, "You know the type."

Alone in the Empty Nest: Clare's Story

A third community type is conveyed in stories of the elderly widow who lives alone in a house that is now too big for her to manage on her own and is located in an area of the city that has lost its former neighborliness. In many ways, this is Rita's story before she moves into public housing to exemplify an altogether different type. In contrast to Rita's thick web of social connections and Ben's useful lack thereof, Clare's story thematizes lost ties, loneliness, and insurmountable difficulties in daily living. It is the story of a woman who thrived on domestic life and local sentiments, who with the aging of the family and changing urban residential patterns finds herself in a totally "empty nest." While the term "empty nest" usually signifies either an aging couple's, widower's, or widow's household in the postparental years, in Clare's case, the type conveys more. Here, the empty nest is not only bereft of children, but also of the social and psychological anchors of home, family living, spousal companionship, and the familiarities of neighborhood. Clare is Polish and has lived all her life in a Polish neighborhood, now no longer Polish.

Of all community types pertaining to frail elderly, this one is perhaps the most vivid in the public consciousness. What it means to grow old in the city is regularly signaled by stories of changing environs, lost ties, and loneliness, not fierce independence or quasi-familial bonds. Clare's story is about the aging widow from virtually any ethnic background whose local community roots have been altered with changing residential patterns. The story is equally about the Italian widow who now lives alone in a neighborhood of Latinos or the elderly black woman who now resides by herself in a neighborhood of Southeast Asians.

A version of Clare's story is told by a community mental health worker, Mark, who has come to know Clare quite well from Clare's frequent visits to the mental health clinic located in a small commercial strip on the main street running by the neighborhood. Mark points out that Clare is not "really mentally ill; she just needs a little support, that's all." In conveying details of Clare's life at present, he explains that because Clare's social world has changed so much in the last few years, she just needs to see that familiar face when she goes out for her walk or to buy the few items needed from the local grocery store. Mark adds that Clare has become increasingly dependent on the mental health clinic and workers for companionship and social support.

The location of the clinic proves difficult for Clare. She has to negotiate a five-block walk through what she repeatedly describes as a scary neighborhood. Clare is 81 years old, suffered a broken hip a few years back, which she has partially recovered from but has some lingering pain, and now walks with increasing difficulty because of the arthritis in her legs and back. This combines with her growing unfamiliarity with the neighborhood's residents to make each local foray a major undertaking.

Clare has four children, who grew up in the neighborhood, went off to college, married, and settled elsewhere. Three live in another state. One resides approximately one hour away by car in a distant suburb. Clare keeps in contact with all of them by telephone. Her husband died at the age of 70; she was 69 then. When he died, what had been an empty nest became an empty house. The 10 or so years since then have been very difficult for her. She misses her children and longs for her husband's companionship.

According to Mark, while Clare now lives by herself and mainly on her own, what makes matters worse for women like her in the later years is that they have had such traditional marriages. In Clare's case, it seems to have been a happy one. But her devotion to housework and homemaking, and her complete reliance on her husband for transportation, financial management, and other common husbandly responsibilities, forms into a lifelong obsolescence. As Mark explains, "She's the type that thrives in a traditional family setting, but when those ties start to loosen, you better watch out." Mark suggests that such ties are the only tradition Clare knows and can comfortably accept, which, under the circumstances, is now a persistent source of trouble.

Clare resists forming ties with her new neighbors, most of whom are not Polish and as Mark reports, "always seem to Clare to want to get things out of her, like borrowing things and not returning them." It is evident that the changed neighborhood has compounded the social isolation established when her children moved away and her husband died. Clare's growing fear of the area, which Mark reports is probably justified to some degree, works to keep her isolated at home, feeding on itself in the process.

Mark points out how in a story such as Clare's, living itself becomes threatening. Clare worries constantly about whether she will be accosted or killed on what she calls "the streets." She fears having an accident at home and lying unconscious on the floor for days with no one to find her. She is anxious that she will die and be left unattended.

As far as intervention is concerned, Mark explains that Clare's is the classic case of a troubled life that one can't do much about because it "falls in the cracks." Clare evidently is adequately housed. While her children are not negligent, neither the children nor Clare can see the possibilty of Clare moving in with any of them. Even though she is in constant pain and has trouble getting about, she is still mobile. She manages some shopping. Other transportation needs are handled for the most part by a local, free van service for the elderly. Although not financially flush, neither is Clare destitute.

According to the mental health worker, in some ways Clare poses more trouble for intervention than the types of frail elderly in the community who are either worse or better off. Loneliness and fright seem to be Clare's greatest difficulties and the most poignant themes of her story. Unfortunately, they are not officially the kinds of trouble a professional worker can do much about. What are very significant troubles for Clare, officially are virtually nonexistent— another version of her story. Certainly, Clare obtains some comfort from visiting the mental health clinic. She has become a familiar face. Most staff members take the time to chat and commiserate with her. Yet all know that it is not enough for her and probably never will be. The life Clare knew, the only life she can imagine fitting into, seems to have passed her by.

The Single, Older Caregiver: Bea's Story

Neugarten (1974) writes that, because substantial numbers of elderly are now living long lives, it is important to distinguish aged persons who are much like the middle-aged from those whose health and social characteristics are more closely associated with the common view of "old." While 65 once was both officially and unofficially considered old age for purposes of retirement, social security benefits, and other markers of later life, it is now clear that being elderly in the years stretching from 55 to 75 or thereabouts offers a dramatic contrast with being elderly, say, from 75 on.

Neugarten refers to those aged 55 to 75 as the "young-old" and those 75 and over as the "old-old." As the segment of the aged population over 85 is the most rapidly growing, it may be necessary in time to revise the old-old category upward, perhaps to 85 and beyond. There is an emerging generation of elderly who themselves precede in years another generation of elderly. While in one sense the distinction is simply demographic in that it separates ranges of years with different vital statistics, in another sense the distinction is highly social and dynamic (Neugarten & Neugarten, 1986). Having two generations of elderly in the same family presents emerging troubles that link directly with the differential ties and traditions of the old-old and the young-old.

It is in this context that Bea's story is considered. As the facilitator of Bea's support group for the family caregivers of Alzheimer's disease victims tells it, Bea's is a special case of the elderly caring for the still older, something "more and more common these days" (Gubrium, 1986a). Bea is 66 years old and cares for her 89-year-old mother at home. The mother has been diagnosed with Alzheimer's disease (senile dementia), is otherwise fairly healthy, and has lucid moments. Bea has plenty of room in her home and, now that she is retired, can ostensibly take all the time required to tend to her mother.

Bea's situation both compares and contrasts with others in the support group. Most are family members of her age or older who care for a demented relative at home. Several are spouses, mainly wives, and are older than Bea. Others, like Bea, are elderly adult children. In certain ways Bea's single status stands out in the support group to make her situation different. Yet, her story is one of a recognizable community type—the spinster on whom the weight of parental care falls completely.

As the group facilitator tells it, Bea is one of the aging breed of women, still around in considerable numbers, who came of marriageable age during World War II. They had boyfriends, were engaged, or were recently married, but their mates were either killed in action or never returned to the same relationship. By mutual agreement, Bea and her boyfriend at the time decided to put off a formal engagement until after the war. The relationship fizzled and Bea never again met a suitable man.

Bea's sisters' and brothers' experiences are different. Two sisters, one older, eventually married and had families of their own. One of two brothers died in action; the other married and never had children. All eventually settled in the same city. None divorced. There are several great grandchildren in the extended family. Bea's sisters are extensively involved in their own adult children's lives. Bea and her childless brother maintain links with nephews and nieces.

Until recently, the extended family has been fairly close knit and its relations cordial. This changed when Bea's father died and her mother's mental demise loomed forth. Bea's marital status as a single person came significantly into play in the family's related dynamics. Bea's particular configuration of ties presented her and her siblings with the sort of trouble none of them, especially Bea, ever imagined would arise.

As the support group facilitator reports, over the years Bea has formed a number of very close ties with other single women. The facilitator describes how often Bea speaks of her friends Molly and Rose. The three have been inseparable confidants for approximately 30 years. None married. Molly lost her fiancee in the war; Rose had never seriously planned to marry. As the facilitator points out, "When you hear Bea talk about them, you'd think she was describing family." But the facilitator also remarks:

> *Things aren't as rosy as they seem. When old Mrs. Calder [Bea's mother] started to forget and to wander, they [Bea and her siblings] decided that the old lady couldn't stay at home. Mrs. Calder had been living alone for years, but evidently her mind was failing. She started to*

*really flip out after her husband died. So they decided to sell the house
and put Mother in one of those adult [congregate] living facilities. Well
that didn't work out. But none of them [the siblings] could think of
placing Mother in a nursing home either. So guess who the lucky one
was? Bea, of course. It's the same old story. Bea doesn't have a family of
her own to take care of, she has the room, and—get this—of course the
brother who doesn't have any children can't take care of Mother because
"you just can't expect a man to do that kind of job."*

The facilitator's comments embellish the story of the typical single elder who seemingly by default cares for a frail elderly
parent. While the facilitator's sarcasm implies that, for her, there is
nothing "natural" about the choice of this family member as a
caregiver, the rest of Bea's story suggests that, to the family members concerned, it is perfectly reasonable and obvious who the home
caregiver should be.

Two things led Bea to the support group. First, when Mrs.
Calder was eventually diagnosed as having Alzheimer's disease, Bea
was attracted to the support group and its affiliation with a local
chapter of the Alzheimer's Disease and Related Disorders Association because the group and chapter promised to be helpful and
convenient sources of information about the disease and its management. Second, Bea's relations with both her siblings and her
close friends—her "two families," she sometimes calls them—became so strained because of her caregiving activity that she needed
to talk with someone sympathetic but not directly involved.

The circumstance of taking in the mother and caring for her
at home causes two separate sets of ties and traditions to clash for
the first time in Bea's life. Until the mother's home care situation is
settled, Bea manages to maintain close ties with both of her "families." Her traditional warm and indulgent relations with her siblings, their children, and the grandchildren are valued by all. She is
"good Aunt Bea." It is taken for granted that Aunt Bea has no family
of her own to gush over. Bea's traditionally intimate and supportive
ties with Molly and Rose are valued too. Even Bea's siblings and
their families love Bea's "dear friends."

In discussing who would take in Mrs. Calder and care for
her, none of the siblings takes serious note of the fact that Bea has

a close "family" (in her friends) who will suffer because of the time and emotional commitments of the new situation. It is assumed that Bea has no family of her own and, thus, is the natural caregiver. This annoys Bea, Molly, and Rose. While, in a way, Bea understands why her siblings think as they do, she is at the same time troubled that none of them give any consideration to the fact that she has close, intimate, and valued ties separate from her siblings and their families. The siblings are surprised and troubled by hints on Bea's part that she is being unfairly imposed upon. Similarly, while in their own ways, Molly and Rose understand the demands placed on Bea by the siblings' expectations and sympathize with Bea's circumstance, the two are distressed by what they see as Bea's deteriorating loyalty to their friendship group. Nor is Bea blind to her two friends' concern and pain, as her comments and tears in the support group indicate.

Still, Bea concludes that, in the final analysis, her troubles are no one's fault in particular. The facilitator remarks that Bea often mentions how "you can't really blame them, can you?" thereby showing that Bea is aware of the circumstance from which everyone's distress arises. Indeed, as the facilitator adds, "She [Bea] keeps saying that if anyone of us were in her place, the same thing would happen." According to the facilitator, however, the trouble this circumstance presents for Bea is that Bea is blaming no one but herself for what is happening. Using a familiar phrase, the facilitator concludes, "You know the story; she doesn't want to hurt anyone—neither of her 'families.' So who gets hurt? Bea, the victim!"

Once more we find that ties, traditions, and troubles work together so that, depending on one's social standpoint, troubles take on different meanings. Bea's is one story told by a single spokesperson, a facilitator. Yet it conveys the versions of its characters' perspectives. Together with Ben's, Rita's, and Clare's stories and the community types they represent, Bea's story complicates community well beyond what the modifier "the" conveys. Each story tells of the multiple meanings of "family," "care," and "caregiving." As Burnley (1987) informs us in her own study of caregiving and single women, and as Gubrium and Holstein (1990) argue in general, caring and responsibility in the real world can only be understood in terms of the various ways family and familial ties are sorted and assigned by those concerned.

Implications for the Professional Caregiver

Just as Frankfather finds that local "stations" cast the community lives of confused elderly in accordance with the stations' respective definitions of trouble, community types and their stories show the wide range of experiences the community can be for frail elderly. While the types described are prominent in the discourse and actions of professional workers, they do not exhaust the diversity. Accurate or not, the phrase "you know the type" references innumerable experiences, from those depicted in the stories of this chapter to the typical elderly widower who lives with his never-married sister, the typical great grandmother who lives isolated and alone in the back room of her grandson's family home, the typical homeless woman who finds shelter and ekes out a living on the streets, the typical black grandmother who lives in the inner city and cares for her daughter's young children, and the typical extended household of the immigrant family where nonEnglish speaking elderly spend their lives. The list, of course, goes on.

Presenting four stories in detail shows, too, that there are diverse ways in which the experience of aging is organized, even within stories. Troubles discerned take on their meaning in accordance with their versions.

DIFFERENCES IN KIND

The variety of differences that is the community has a bearing on planning and intervention. For example, one cannot expect that an elderly man or woman who is about to reenter the community after a stint in a health care facility will necessarily enter a domain whose characteristics are simply opposite to those found in institutions. One will not necessarily be without the support a facility provides. One may in fact find oneself in the midst of something more elaborate, as Rita's circumstances show. On the other hand, one will not necessarily return to family and friends. One may in fact find oneself virtually bereft of both the familial and the communal in the midst of a neighborhood, as Clare's story suggests.

To approach the community as the simple opposite of what might be equally stereotyped *the* institution is a polarity that requires specification in practice. It is not that the polarity is useless; it does, after all, inform us that care needs and caregiving are a range of circumstances and options, as the idea of a continuum of care suggests. Yet, at the same time, the polarity, like the idea of a linear continuum of care, implies that there is a linking thread underlying the options—alternatives in degree, not in kind. One polarity is more or less of the other. In contrast, practice shows that the specification of community living depends on the type of experience said to comprise it. In this context, we find that there are differences in kind, not degree, according with the particular life stories of members. When we take types and their stories into account, the community is unnumerably distinct experiences.

IMPOSING LINEAR THINKING

Planning and mounting interventions as if these differences did not exist results in linear thinking and the imposition of service-oriented models onto life experiences that are multifaceted, disjointed, and often contradictory. Ignoring types, their stories, and versions is tantamount to taking one story, building a general model of needs, care, and intervention from it and approaching all types of experiences in the community in terms of it.

BALANCING THEORY AND THE REAL WORLD

Theory and the real world must be kept in constant balance. Unfortunately, there are opposing forces. The professionalization of caregiving, for one, has a tendency to place theory (models, systems) at the center of planning and organized intervention. Certification and licensing compel the professional caregiver to show special conceptual and procedural competence. Regulating and funding agencies circumscribe the formal design of caregiving plans and activities. The result is that the caregiving experience becomes the handmaiden of theory rather than its partner. This is why the real world is such an eye-opener for the neophyte and why it is difficult for anyone to negotiate.

CHAPTER 3

The Home Care Experience

Long-term care is commonly associated with institutionalization, in particular the nursing home. Other care settings—the hospital, the rehabilitation facility, the geriatric clinic—contrast in offering relatively short-term stays. At the same time, the home is becoming an important component of the health care system. The high costs of institutionalization have combined with the growing population of frail elderly, the availability of transportable care apparatus, and the development of a home care industry to bring the household into realistic focus as a care setting.

The emerging significance of the home as a care setting is taking place against a background of heightened debate over familial obligations. As several commentators note (Poster, 1978; Donzelot, 1979; Lasch, 1979), the terms "family," "household," "home," and "filial responsibility" are anything but neutral references to domestic life. They are as much political slogans as they feature domestic relations. On the right, they convey traditional values of home life, which underscore the obligation of family members to secure the whole, as oppressive as the latter might be. On the left, they just as readily hearken patriarchy, domination, and exclusion, even while this might secure domestic order. Despite contrasting political preferences, ideal sentiments of house, home, and familial responsibility attract all. The harsh realities of family living notwithstanding, the home is believed to be the preferred context for coming of age and growing old (Gubrium & Holstein, 1990). As far as elderly are concerned, ideally the family safeguards its own, as it were, as the later years take their toll of body and mind.

Yet, as Gubrium and Sankar (1990) note, while there is much public discussion and debate about the home, family, and home care and continuing development of related professional activity, the home is only dimly understood as a "sickroom" (Rubinstein, 1990). We know little about its interpersonal dynamics and culture as the setting for practical activities centered on caregiving. There are a number of important questions for which answers are needed. What is the meaning of familial responsibility to those concerned? How do families learn what they are, and are not, responsible for in caring for frail elderly at home? How do those involved evaluate, in their own terms, the quality of home care? How much caregiving is enough? What kind of care is sufficient? Indeed, what does it mean to "care" in the first place? How do the traditional sentiments and interpersonal ties of the family enter into, and shape, members' sense of responsibility? While this chapter does not consider all the questions, it does explore their underlying real-world dynamic.

The Care Equation

The modeling, measurement, and assessment of family members' home care has become a virtual research industry. For about 10 years, social, behavioral, and health care scientists have attempted to study the relationship between what originally were three caregiving factors: the frail elderly family members' level of impairment; the family caregiver's felt burden or stress; and the likelihood of institutionalization. This increasingly has centered on the home care of Alzheimer's disease victims. (The disease can manifest itself mainly in dementia or be combined with physical frailties and other debilities of old age.) A quick look at recent proceedings of annual conferences of the Gerontological Society of America shows that an initial three-factor model has grown into complex configurations of primary and intervening variables.

The original home *care equation* is grounded in deceptively straightforward reasoning. Center stage is the family caregiver, usually elderly and female, who cares for an increasingly frail elder in the home. Focal is the "burden," "felt burden," "stress," or "strain" of caregiving. Both subjective and objective sides are distinguished. In an early study, Zarit, Reever, and Bach-Peterson (1980) refer to the subjective side as the "felt burden" and assess it by means of a 29-item, self-report inventory administered to the primary caregiver. Poulshock and Deimling (1984) later tap into objective aspects such as the caregiver's estimate of how personally tiring, difficult, or upsetting the impairments are. Poulshock and Deimling further distinguish the subjective and objective burden from what they call the personal "impact" of the burden of care—the material and social consequences of caregiving—such as the resulting financial difficulties and familial disruptions.

In the original reasoning, as the care receiver's impairment worsens, it presents an increasing burden of care to the caregiver, which, in turn, affects the caregiver's tolerance, eventually requiring the care receiver's institutionalization. Overall, the model is framed negatively: one bad thing leads to another. There is little or no sense that, for some caregivers or family members, the impairment might not be conceived as a burden nor, for that matter, institutionalization meaningfully entertained. Reflecting Lewis and Meredith's linear thinking, the care equation urges adherents to interpret the meaning of home care in relation to a continuum of options with the household at one end and the nursing home at the other.

With a particular image of caregiving at the forefront, original input and output variables are clear. The input is the care receiver's impairment. Emphasizing the negative, the idea is that the care receiver's condition is poor and getting worse, not that he or she simply ages (Gubrium & Lynott, 1987). There is no sense that the changing mental and physical conditions of old age as they bear on the family might be, for some members and caregivers, the converse of the changing mental and physical conditions of growing up, to be accepted as natural. Rather, as Zarit, Orr, and Zarit (1985) imply in the title of their guide for caregivers, "families under stress" are thought to be "hidden *victims* of Alzheimer's disease" (emphasis added).

The output is the institutionalization decision, in particular the question of whether to seek nursing home placement. Again the emphasis is on the negative. In the original thinking, the impairment eventually becomes so burdensome and the stress so severe that the only alternative is institutional care. The idea of a continuum of care supports this reasoning, specifying the nursing home as the solution of choice when all else fails. The refusal to seek institutionalization is thought itself to be a kind of sickness called "denial" (Gubrium, 1988b). Again, there is no notion that families might define care in both the short- and long-run as an ordinary domestic matter.

Since its original formulation, the care equation has been embellished to include a number of intervening variables and in the process, the priority of its three original components, altered. One of the first intervening variables considered is social support, stemming from the question of whether expressed concern or expressions of help for the caregiver lessens felt strain and the likelihood of the care receiver's institutionalization. Zarit, Reever, and Bach-Peterson (1980) and later Zarit, Orr, and Zarit (1985) show that an informal support network, such as regular visits and expressions of support from relatives, mitigate the effect of an overwhelming burden on the home caregivers of Alzheimer's disease victims. Morycz (1985) finds that back-up help and the victim's marital status affect the desire to seek institutionalization. Deimling and Poulshock (1985) report that factors such as the caregiver's precrisis attitude toward the suitability of nursing home care and the personal well-being of the caregiver are important ingredients in figuring the likelihood of institutionalization.

What emerges is a greater awareness of the need to consider the *meaning* of the care equation's factors to those concerned. Still, a "linear" view predominates. Summarizing the results of the research in this area, Gwyther and George (1986) stress the complications that a broad range of intervening variables impose on the original care equation. They conclude (1) that the caregiver's felt burden depends on the caregiver's relationship with the care receiver and (2) the receiver's impairment is relatively insignificant for understanding the caregiver's functioning. The upshot is that the priority of the impairment is reduced and the caregiver's social situation emphasized. They do not question the linear view and the language is still negative, linking together the ideas of burden, stress, strain, and caregiver tolerance.

The Care Experience

___

A small but growing body of research is taking exception to this way of thinking (Gubrium & Lynott, 1987; Gubrium & Sankar, 1990). Echoing Lewis & Meredith's (1988) sentiments, the research suggests that the native experiences of caregiving are more realistically captured when a linear, service-oriented framework is set aside and replaced by a view toward caregiving's complex and dynamic relationships. Lewis and Meredith caution that the framework directly or implicitly chosen to organize studies has its own way of interpreting social facts, separate from what the facts themselves indicate.

On both sides of the Atlantic, sociologists and anthropologists are heeding advice of this sort and studying the *care experience*, that is, how those involved in home care frame and interpret it. The research is qualitative. Some studies are based on intensive, open-ended interviews with caregivers (Burnley, 1987; Rubinstein, 1990; Wenger, 1987), some on participant observation in the home (Sankar, 1986, 1988), others on household interviews and participant observation in settings outside the home where caregivers share the meaning of home care (Gubrium, 1986a, 1988b; Gubrium & Lynott, 1987; Holstein, 1990), and still others on a combination of qualitative methods (Jerrome, 1983; Gubrium & Sankar, 1990). Their common point of reference is the understanding that the study of caregiving must be grounded in the real world in the actual, lived experience or interpretive practices of those concerned (Glaser & Strauss, 1967; Gubrium, 1988a).

ASSUMPTIONS OF CARE EXPERIENCE STUDIES

Four assumptions underpin studies of the home care experience.

Nothing inevitable. First, it is assumed that there is nothing inevitable about the realtionship between impairment, caregiving, and institutionalization. One thing does not naturally lead to another, no matter how complicated the relationship is by other variables. Whatever those directly involved in, or attendant to, caregiving taken for granted is considered to be natural.

Experiential learning. It is assumed that the meaning of the caregiving experience is learned. This draws attention to the learning process. A number of important questions arise in this regard: From whom and where does the caregiver learn to perceive the impairment as, say, a burden or strain? Do caregivers sometimes learn to perceive the impairment differently? What circumstances bear on the learning process? Do caregivers perceive the home care situation in terms of burden in one circumstance and in terms of, say, filial loyalty, in another? What is the social organization of the learning? Are there more or less well-established learning "programs," as it were? For example, do service agents or agencies "teach" caregivers who come into contact with them different ways to view the care experience? Frankfather's (1977) work on community stations is suggestive here.

Meaning assembled. Another assumption is that the meaning of caregiving is assembled and assigned. The history of familial relationships is particularly significant here. What the caregiver presently makes of the impairment is embedded in his or her past relationship with the care receiver. Caregivers do not simply judge their activity as, say, more or less burdensome. Among other biographical considerations, judgments are affected by the interpersonal tradition of affection between the caregiver and care receiver.

Not necessarily negative or positive. Fourth, no ingredient of the home care experience is necessarily either negative or positive. While the care equation frames its components in a language of deficits and last resorts, studies of the care experience assume that any component may be assigned positive or negative meanings, even not given much thought at all. For example, a caregiver may take pride in managing a frail elder at home and in achieving the semblance of a job well done. Another caregiver may take pleasure in the company of someone constantly in the home, frailty notwithstanding. This, of course, does not suggest that there are no naturally occurring, negative sentiments.

In sum, in order to understand the care experience, it is important to take account of the diverse and sundry meanings that caregiving can have, on the one hand, and how the meanings are organized, on the other. Two stories shed light on the complications.

Quality of Care: Harry's Story

Nursing homes, hospitals, and other facilities are regularly evaluated for their quality of care. Consumers of formal care and professional workers seeking placement for clients take note of related criteria of good care. Checklists of "what to look for" or "what a family needs to know" are available for selecting a nursing home. Johnson and Grant's (1985) informative book about the nursing home in American society presents a sample checklist. Three essential points are:

1. Be assured that the nursing home and its administrator have a current state license.
2. If the patient needs financial assistance and if he or she is eligible for government or other forms of assistance, select a home that is certified to participate in the program.
3. For the patient requiring a special diet or specific type of therapy, make certain that the home can provide the needed services. (p. 120)

The authors, of course, list other things to take into account, from the safety of the physical plant, to cleanliness, the provision of activity programs, and staffing characteristics. In general, checklists combine standards drawn from regulatory agencies with items of public interest.

It is difficult to imagine how such standards might apply to home care. Even while the home is emerging as an important site for the long-term care of the elderly, the home's informality, spontaneity, and privacy seem to preclude standards and checklists. Yet families, elderly, and professional workers do take account of what is happening in the home—both the home's offerings and their quality—in assigning meaning and value to the home care experience. Harry's story is a foil to the custom of thinking about quality of care in terms of *formal* care organization. As Harry's story shows, the quality of home care is far from a simple matter of the degree of burden an impairment presents or the extent of a surrounding support network. Quality is mediated by ties, traditions, and troubles.

Harry's story comes from a study of the descriptive organization of dementia (Gubrium, 1986a). He has been visiting a local geriatric clinic and occasionally participates in the clinic's support program for family caregiver's of Alzheimer's disease victims. Harry and his wife, Ruth, are in their eighties, have been married for 60 years, and have three sons. The sons have professional careers, families of their own, and live in different regions of the country. While Ruth's condition has been diagnosed Alzheimer's, she had a number of age-related disorders before the onset of dementia. To Harry, she suffers as much from the latter as she does from the dementia. The dementia is just one more insult to what has been a very dear, loving, and charmed relationship. Ruth is confined to a wheelchair, is lucid at times, occasionally incontinent, and cared for in their apartment by her husband. They live alone, as they have for the many years since their youngest son left home.

Harry still drives and manages on his own to visit the geriatric clinic when he needs to consult a nurse or physician about his wife or to infrequently participate in its family program. He prefers the company of the elderly men and women who attend a local church's day program because, according to Harry, it is friendlier and less regimented than the geriatric clinic's offerings. Harry and Ruth are Jewish.

Harry's story has many versions. Staff members at the clinic have a view of his home care situation. A facilitator at the support group Harry occasionally attends in the Jewish Community Center has a version. Harry has his own account. There are others. Taking account of the many tellings suggests that the quality of his home care has many interpretations. I will not detail each of them, but focus on a few as points of contrast.

Dora, an employee of the geriatric clinic, has been acquainted with Harry for years, even before he became active in the clinic's programs. She remembers when Ruth was an able and lively 75-year-old:

Those two? They're like, well, egg and yolk; you can't separate them. They've always been like that, all the time I've known them. She was always the lively and poised little lady. Harry's got a sharp tongue and tells it like it is. When it comes to Ruth, well he's her guardian and hovers around her. He really dotes on her. No one can say anything that's even a little bit critical or they'll hear it from Harry. There's just nothing she could ever do wrong. He's still the same, even though I don't think she really recognizes him anymore. That doesn't seem to faze him. I think a lot of the trouble he's having is connected to the fact that he refuses to recognize that.

After Dora makes the necessary arrangements, I visit Harry and Ruth in their apartment. Harry greets me at the door and enthusiastically remarks that he has been looking forward to my coming because, as he puts it, "I don't often get a visit from a professional man and I have lots and lots of time for that." Harry is most solicitous, inviting me in and offering me the best chair in the room.

Harry's enthusiasm is founded on an old and deep respect for learning. He did not have the opportunity to get much formal education beyond high school. He has thrived in the clothing business. He and Ruth made every effort to see that their sons were well educated. The pride he takes in his sons, their training, and their professional success is evident. Harry himself commands a good informal education, speaking with ease and surprising erudition about many things, from current events to the present state of the medical establishment.

The enthusiasm seems to be dampened by the gloom of the caregiving scene that surrounds us. As Harry and I talk, his wife, who is seated in a wheelchair in the middle of the room, occasionally mumbles or grunts incomprehensibly. Harry attends to her periodically, checking for an episode of incontinence or otherwise adjusting her body in the chair from the slumping, crooked position it has assumed. The room smells of urine. I find the room too warm, in fact, stifling. Harry mentions the urine odor and the heat, as well as the general messiness of the apartment. I have not yet taken notice of the mess. But he dismisses them as "the kinds of things that come with the territory," as he puts it, meaning that the conditions are a normal part of home care. He adds with emphasis that, in any case, there are more important things to think about—like how Ruth feels, what she needs, and the things he has to do to take good care of her. This is the first time Harry mentions what amounts to a statement about the quality of home care.

I have several more visits with Harry. We have long and touching conversations. It becomes clear that, for Harry, the quality of home care is linked to entirely different considerations than it is for Dora and others. Harry and I talk about matters reminiscent of the care equation, discussing Ruth's impairments, the stresses and strains of home care, the burden of managing someone incontinent and wheelchair-bound, and the condition of nursing homes in the vicinity and the nation at large. I witness Harry monitoring Ruth at home, transporting her to and from the apartment, negotiating her frail body into and out of his car, conversing with her in a way Harry claims to be meaningful, affectionately holding her and tenderly touching her face and hair, and smiling warmly when Ruth moves, among a host of cares and persistent caring. I also witness expressions of frustration associated with the activities.

Whatever Harry says about stress, strain, burden, and impairment, and however extended the frustrations, it becomes evident, too, that, for Harry, these exist at the margins of caregiving. When he speaks of Ruth's impairments, they are not defined as interpersonally burdensome. Rather, they are burdens one encounters in the process of tending to bodily needs. Yes, Ruth's inability to walk makes it difficult for Harry to get Ruth from place to place. Yes, her incontinence makes it hard to keep their surroundings odorless and neat. Yes, her inability to communicate at times frustrates his attempt to efficiently fulfil her ostensible desires. But these are more or less burdensome as tasks; they do not prevail on his motivation to continue caring for her tenderly and to keep her as close to him and as comfortable as possible.

There are two different senses of burden implied, which, for Harry, are not connected. As his testimony and sentiments indicate, one is merely instrumental, the other relational. As far as the instrumental burden is concerned, the quality of Harry's care reflects elements of the care equation. In speaking about and commenting on his caregiving activities, Harry links Ruth's growing frailty with the strain of caring for her. Her bodily ills and her "dimming, but once bright mind" get in the way of attending to her. He occasionally makes overtures to the desirability of having home help, comparing that with all that might be done for Ruth in an institutional setting. Harry reports that he sometimes thinks about how his own effort to care for Ruth at home might be cheating her of what professional caregivers could more effectively do.

The link drawn between the impairments, the burden of care, the strain, and professional care does not extend to Harry and Ruth's interpersonal relationship. That is categorically separate, having an entirely different meaning and quality. As Harry states many times, "That there, my friend, is something else altogether." It is not a matter of burden, stress, strain, or disengagement at all.

Harry reminds me that Ruth is "the world" to him and, in this regard, she can "never, never be a burden." He once mentions that every time he "strains" or pushes himself "to the limit" in caring for her, he knows she senses how much he loves her and that makes him glad to be her spouse, as if to inform me that stress and strain can have a positive outcome.

The straightforward application of the care equation confounds an important experiential distinction. Harry's comments and activities show that as far as caregiving is concerned, he is tied to Ruth in at least two ways. The quality of his home care reflects the complication. His instrumental tie with her in caregiving causes him considerable trouble. He contemplates what someone with more training, or a facility with additional services, might offer. In this regard, the quality of Harry's home care admittedly leaves something to be desired. Harry's interpersonal tie with Ruth, however, is an entirely different matter for him, not conceived in terms of trouble. Interpersonally, he has a vivid and passionate tradition of loyalty and gratitude, which both informs him of the meaning of and secures his commitment to his wife's home care. When it comes to that, Harry accepts all the "trouble" required to make Ruth happy and comfortable. In this context, there is little doubt in Harry's mind that the quality of his care is impeccable.

The different experiential linkages of burden, stress, and strain are not unique to Harry's home care experience. Other caregivers make similar distinctions in their stories of home care. For them, the care experience is a mosaic of two kinds of story—one a tale of daily woe and the other a narrative of total commitment. Of course, not all caregivers' experiences have these characteristics. At one extreme are the few who resolutely refuse to entertain any burden, stress, and strain at all, even of an instrumental kind. At the other extreme are those who see the quality of home care in totally instrumental terms, telling their stories accordingly.

The professional service providers working with Harry and other family caregivers combine these distinct domains of experience into the view of a single, linear caregiving adjustment process. This is reflected in Dora's version of the quality of Harry's home care experience. Her thoughts are decidedly at odds with Harry's view. She sees a stage-like process of adjustment in home care, which is informed by a larger and emerging public culture of elderly home care. Indeed, the larger understanding provides a framework for family caregivers within which to judge their own thoughts and feelings. Harry is among the exceptions, refusing to entertain the broader framework in relation to his own experience.

The public culture of the Alzheimer's disease movement portrays the caregiver's adjustment as coming in stages (Gubrium, 1986a, 1986b, 1988b). From broadcast media, caregiver handbooks, newsletters, popular literature, informational films, support groups, and local chapters of the Alzheimer's Disease and Related Disorders Association (ADRDA), the received wisdom is that at first family members are understandably concerned with cure and recovery. The caregiver zeros in on whatever can be used to eliminate or, at least, slow the progress of the illness. There is a decided press for news of medical developments, so-called breakthroughs in cure. The caregiver's own well-being remains in the background. Accordingly, in describing the changing reactions of caregivers who visit her geriatric clinic or participate in its support group, Dora regularly explains that one can tell the novices because they seem always to care more about the patient than themselves.

A second stage of adjustment is entered as the caregiver begins to have doubts about the possibility of recovery. While family members who come into contact with the disease's public culture repeatedly hear that Alzheimer's is a disease with no known cause or cure, this typically is initially taken to be a message about the disease in general, not its status in individual patients. In some disease manifestations, cognitive decline and accompanying physical deficits are not as rapid nor as extensive as in others. Caregivers and families are reminded that a definitive diagnosis of the disease can be made only at autopsy, underscoring the possibility that what happens in individual cases might not reflect what, in theory, is the disease's inevitable progress. It is frequently stated that there is considerable individual variation in the disease's onset and course (Gubrium, 1987b). When the caregiver wonders whether his or her own afflicted family member is exceptional, the second stage is evident.

A third stage comes when the caregiver begins to consider seriously the daily personal stress and strain that the care burden imposes. Caregivers who come into contact with the disease's public culture regularly hear that the disease presents "36-hour" daily burdens (Mace & Rabins, 1981). In the face of this, the so-called realistic caregiver turns primary attention away from the patient's cure and recovery to his or her own well-being. By "denying" the inevitable, those refusing to make the adjustment risk becoming what is said to be the disease's second victim. In time, however, most caregivers, family members, and significant others ostensibly realize that the well-being of the family at large is at risk in continued home care and that the care option of choice is the nursing home.

A fourth stage is sometimes distinguished, applicable to those who have institutionalized a frail, elderly family member. While the characteristics of this stage are not as clear as the others, its experiences entail the mixed emotions of guilt and justification, the result of having placed a loved one in a nursing home. In theory, successful resolution of this stage completes the process of adjustment.

Dora's interpretation of the quality of Harry's home care reflects this linear model. While Dora knows in considerable detail what transpires in Harry's home, his coping style and history, and the course of Ruth's afflictions, Dora does not view the situation in terms of Harry's complex ties with his frail wife. Dora sees Harry as refusing to realize that continued home care, under the circumstances, means a looming crisis in the mental and physical health of all who are directly involved, in particular, Ruth and Harry. As Dora puts it, Harry's is "the familiar story" of the caregiver who doesn't want to see that the situation is hopeless and that, for the caregiver's own good, life must go on. She has remarked on several occasions that Harry is "in that stage" of denial, just before "they" begin to realize that their own and other family members' health is as important as the patient's. Dora explains that each time she advises Harry to consider nursing home placement, which, she adds, Harry can afford, he refuses to listen. Her version of Harry's story takes the continuum of care as the ultimate prescription for his troubles, glossing over the native complications of Harry's own sense of the quality of his relationship with Ruth in caregiving.

From Dora's point of view, Harry's established ties with Ruth, in the current circumstance, are disastrous. As Dora cautions, "That situation is a royal road to hell for everyone concerned." According to Dora, the ties do, and will continue to, present myriad troubles for Harry and Ruth. What is more, according to Dora, the children will feel increasingly pressured to intervene while, at the same time, be reluctant to interfere. From Dora's point of view, for the sake of all concerned, it is time to break out of what she takes to be a perilous tradition of devotion—for everyone's sake.

Whether or not Dora's interpretation is accepted as truth, it is nonetheless her informed evaluation of the situation. Her sense of the quality of care is as much a product of the public culture circumscribing her interpretation of Harry's ties and troubles as it is based in fact. What Dora and other professional workers hold in theory provides a sense of the facts in its own right.

The History of Ties: Sally's Story

The care receiver's impairment, the caregiver's response, social support, and the question of institutionalization commonly are evaluated in terms of how they presently impinge on the lives of those concerned, using what Lewis and Meredith (1988) call a "snapshot" approach. Yet caregiving stories show that the present meaning of experience has enduring connections with the past and the future. How does the history of ties between the caregiver and care receiver enter into the meaning of the caregiving relationship?

Sally's story suggests that the mosaic of care constituting the real world is, in a manner of speaking, long told. She is the 68-year-old caregiver for her 90-year-old elderly mother, Carmen, who has Alzheimer's disease. Sally cares for Carmen at home. As Carmen's forgetfulness and demands worsen, Sally tells of increasing strain, especially resentment. Yet the effects are not directly related to her mother's impairment. As Sally points out, "If it was just the caregiving, the hands-on stuff, I'd have it made." Sally explains that she has as much time as she needs to care for her mother.

The strain and resentment have to do with her life-long mixed feelings for her mother, a part of their relationship ever since she was a "little girl," she repeats both in conversations at home and in her support group. In a long afternoon discussion at home, Sally describes how "mother is when she gets really bad," tellingly tying this to old feelings.

> Sometimes—you saw some of it the last time we talked—she [her mother] just gets very upset with herself. She'll be real good all morning and then, snap, she gets real sulky and starts to demand things. I know

right away something's wrong. Most of the time, I know she's probably messed in her pants or something. She's gotten worse lately and, to say the least, it's difficult. I usually don't mind that kind of stuff, really . . . I raised a lot of kids and now I take care of my grandchildren. I've seen a lot of dirty diapers in my time. It's not that. Well, it's just that, well, she starts to yell, and demands, and as I'm cleaning her up, those old feelings come up again—like when I was a little girl.

Another day, again in Sally's home, she recalls what it was like for her when she was a little girl growing up with her mother. This prompts Sally's husband to chide Sally for repeating a story he has heard time and again, at which she scoffs and continues. The old feelings that now make it difficult to deal with her mother's impairment involve a particular mixture of life-long resentment and love.

Sally at first cryptically explains that what she feels is "different," as she puts it, from what her sisters and brothers feel. Speaking about her two older brothers, Sally then elaborates. She describes their achievements glowingly, telling how her parents, especially her mother, encouraged their success. Sally has been proud of them, too. But she resents how the encouragement and success readily combined for them; she feels it hasn't in her own case. While in Sally's opinion, she has been a successful homemaker, it was not the result of her mother's encouragement. Sally speaks similarly about her two younger sisters, who were the family "babies," particularly the youngest: "When I was a little girl, I just resented how they [the parents], especially my mother, doted on those two; sometimes it's like I didn't exist." As with the brothers, Sally mentions how much she has admired her sisters, who, like herself, have been successful homemakers and raised fine children.

Sally places these life-long feelings in the context of caring for her mother. She explains that whenever she thinks about how differently she was treated by her mother, her otherwise positive feelings about her brothers seem to "turn sour," especially now that the entire burden of caring for their mother has been placed on her. The same mixture of resentment and love extends to her sisters, except that in their case Sally resents that she was not "babied" as they were.

The complications provide an unfortunate set of troubles for Sally, both in relations with her mother and her siblings. Sally is acutely aware of this. She blames herself for the troubles *she* causes at times. This is apparent in the following comments Sally makes in a support group meeting.

> *When I think about it . . . and I have a habit of really, really thinking about it too much sometimes . . . I just get myself all worked up. Like things will be going along real nice-like with them [her brothers and sisters] and, then, I'll start to think about how they got all the attention when we were growing up . . . like Mother thought those two [younger sisters] were little Kewpie dolls. [Elaborately describes the mother's indulgence of her sisters.] It was just god-awful sometimes. It made me sick to think about it and it still makes me sick. [Describes her reaction at length.] Well, it shows; I just know Mary and Bev [the sisters] sense it and they start to react. You can just see what it leads to. They start to give me the cold shoulder and I just get madder and madder inside. It causes a lot of trouble. But that's family life, I guess.*

Sally describes how she tries to deal with the problem of the past "creeping out," as she puts it, and affecting her present relations with her mother and siblings.

> *It's something that's hard to control. You do have a past and you just can't forget what it was. It seems that no matter how hard you try, you remember what it was like and that colors how you feel now. What I try to do is to keep my mind on what each of them means to me. Like my husband says, "Keep it simple." You try to forget the past. I tell myself, "What Mother felt and how she acted is one thing and what Mary and Bev and the boys [her brothers] are to me is something else." That helps to keep things sorted out. But, you know, it's hard to control those old feelings, things you always were to each other. You just can't turn it off like a faucet.*

Tradition is a force of its own, which Sally tries to contain by sorting historical linkages, something she finds difficult.

In describing her thoughts and feelings in caring for her mother, Sally poignantly indicates how the history of affections concretely enters into the present, emphasizing, "It's worse than it might appear."

You know, you do the kinds of things you have to. When she messes up, I just hunker down and clean it up and clean her up too. You can get real close when that kind of thing happens; I mean real close. Think about it. There's your mother—you know the one who wiped your behind when you were a kid and carried you around naked and who you never, never thought needed help and you never, never saw her naked. God forbid! And here she is looking up at you all exposed and helpless and you're wiping her. She's confused and hardly knows it's you sometimes. She's so helpless. Thinking about it makes me want to cry. God bless her. But then, I think, "Why am I feeling this way when she never really gave me a second thought if Mary or Bev or the boys were around?" You start to resent her and all the trouble she's causing in your life. That really makes it all the much harder. Believe me, it's worse than it might appear. Think about it—try to care for someone when naked flesh is pressed to totally naked flesh that you resent and love and ask yourself how you'd feel.

The past is not a mere fixture in its impact on the present; it has a way of oscillating into and out of Sally's estimation of the burden she carries. At one point in a support group session, she makes a telling comment in this regard. While she believes her support group offers her the opportunity to vent her feelings, participants' advice to her is sometimes as troublesome as the troubles they are meant to help alleviate. In response to several participants' comparisons of the burdens they experience in caring for an incontinent Alzheimer's patient at home and their suggestions about forgetting the past, Sally remarks:

I really don't think it's that simple, not for me anyway. Like I was saying about trying to keep the past in the past. When I'm able to do that, I just feel very fond of Mother. It can be very close and I feel very close. At those times, no matter how much bother she is, I don't feel she's a burden really. I feel that, well, she's my mother and I love her. You don't think much of it [the burden of care], really. But watch out when you start to think back! I have a bad habit of doing that. It can creep up on you . . . just like that. [Snaps her fingers.] You have to get a hold of yourself, "I just can't take this anymore; it's just too much on me." You resent it and resent it, and . . . you start to resent the fact that you feel the way you do and the burden of that [the resentment] makes it that much worse. Of course, it's not always like that. Just sometimes.

Such oscillations in the place of tradition and ties in everyday life are too complicated to be understood in terms of a care equation. As Abel (1989) concludes from her own ethnographic material about daughters caring for mothers, the history of relationships can affect the recent past and current period in complex ways, the ignorance of which shortchanges the understanding of what it presently means to care for someone. Sally's story shows that the care experience can shift the burden of care, stress, and strain from one extreme to another in a matter of moments. In a half-hour period, it is possible for the caregiver first to perceive him- or herself as extensively burdened by the cares of an impaired family member and then hardly to recognize the mere "bother" the concrete details of caregiving entailed earlier. The fluctuation of an interpersonal tradition in time produces its own shifting versions.

Implications for the Professional Caregiver

These stories have the following implications for the professional caregiver.

DYNAMIC AND COMPLEX LINKAGES

Rigidly conceived variables, formulated in a care equation, cannot capture the dynamic categorical linkages that exist both inside and outside the immediate experience of care. Harry's story informs us that what are commonly considered to be coinciding conditions internal to the personal experience of caregiving—felt burden, stress, strain, and care commitment—can be diametrically opposed. Harry's "burden" is bothersome but otherwise marginal to his devoted concern for his frail wife. Dora, the professional worker in Harry's story, brings a linear image to the interpretation of his caregiving to depict a husband not responding healthily to his grossly impaired spouse. According to Dora, Harry is failing to make a normal transition from dwelling on the care receiver to concern for the caregiver's personal well-being. Sally's past relations with her mother, notably her perception of the mother's differential treatment of her children, are an historical source of Sally's present sense of burden in her mother's care, both ebbing and flowing in its impact on Sally's feelings about the most concrete details of daily care.

Ties, traditions, and troubles differentially complicate the meaning of home care. When Harry thinks of his ties with Ruth in terms of concrete needs and instrumental obligations, she is indeed "a whole lot of trouble," as Harry put it. But this is not the only tie to Ruth that interprets his relations with her. For Harry, it is only the leanest link in a more profound connection. In contrast, Dora's linear, stage-oriented view of the caregiver's adjustment deceptively simplifies the complications to cast as unidimensional what Harry takes to be differences in kind.

The dynamic and complex linkages suggest that what some take as general to the caregiving experience is, in practice, only a version of it. The professional caregiver who does not critically reflect on how he or she frames experience, stands to encounter troubles that will not go away because they derive from the professional's own understanding of caregiving. In part, Harry's situation bothers Dora because Dora conceives of Harry as troubled in a way he does not. The stage-like image of caregiver adjustment guiding Dora's approach and intervention produces its own brand of troubles. As long as Dora is steadfast in this view, the trouble remains and is likely to worsen as the parties involved interact.

MISCONSTRUING MALADJUSTMENT

The professional worker who does not see that the client's social relations have long and enduring pasts misconstrues the complications of the present for caregiver maladjustment. While a professional worker's version of Sally's story was not presented, the facilitator of the support group Sally attends did consider Sally to be confused at times about her relations with her mother and advised Sally to forget the past. Discussion of Sally's situation in the group shows that the term "confusion" referred to the unfortunate state of Sally's mind, not the biographical complications of her present situation.

When Sally's troubles are personalized, she is presented with an admonitory burden in its own right, challenged to recover from her confusion by what amounts to advice to straighten out her thoughts and feelings. She is urged to buy into the model of caregiver adjustment prevalent in the local culture of the support group, which is corroborated by the broader public culture of the disease experience. Following advice to forget the past and to think only of the present and the future, it is pointed out that if Sally does not eventually forget the present, too, and concentrate on the future—namely, the future of her own well-being—the past will cast a very long shadow on the rest of her life. Sally tries to do just that by attempting to repress her resentment.

But it is a temporary solution, for Sally knows in her own way that what her mother, siblings, and family life now mean to her is bound to its historical understanding. To forget the past is not only to resolve mixed feelings but simultaneously to cast doubt on the fact that she is the daughter of this particular mother and sibling to these brothers and sisters. An entire complex of roles and relations is at risk.

The professional worker might consider that the personalization of troubles with deep historical connections might be adding fuel to the fire. In Sally's case, it is possible that she not only would continue to be burdened by the combined resentment and love she experiences in intimately caring for her mother, but further burdened by an intervention that treats her as solely responsible for her current troubles.

THE UPSIDE OF CAREGIVING

While the care equation frames the home care experience in negative terms, the mosaic of care indicates caregiving has its upside, too. Harry's story, for one, shows that he derives considerable pleasure from caring for Ruth. He states that if he can just remain able to do all the little things it takes to keep Ruth on an "even keel" and reasonably happy, he would have done the greatest thing he could for her and be glad about it. Thus, it is entirely possible that caregivers reap pleasure from caring.

In this regard, it is important that the professional worker be alert to the language in which the family caregiver presents the home care experience. While some do convey it in terms of the care equation, others consider the care experience to be an achievement, not a burden. Care is not something to be managed, contained, and ultimately displaced by another, more "realistic" attitude. The point, of course, is not that the home care experience is not negative, but that it can be termed positively.

The two stories of this chapter do not represent the entire mosaic of home care. There are stories in which estimates of the future, too, figure in the interpretation of the present. As Sally, Harry, and others consider what it would mean to institutionalize the care receiver or continue to care for him or her at home, what is foreseen takes its toll of existing relations and understandings. For some, the portent of institutionalization signals welcome, albeit remorseful, relief. For others, it spells the conclusion of a personal responsibility. For still others, it harbors the fear of loneliness.

CHAPTER 4

The Question of Institutionalization

Reckoned by clock time, the past is long gone and the future is yet to come. The present is here and now. As far as our daily affairs are concerned, the present is what matters, should be dealt with, and instructs the realism of actions and decisions. Yet, as Sally's story indicated, in the real world the past has a way of continually creeping into the present, even at a distance of 50 or 60 years. The past not only comes forth, but without it the sum and substance of what lives continue to be can be lost. The experiential meaning of things in time flows backward just as much as it runs ahead. It bends on itself so that the future runs parallel to the past and serves as a basis of comparison, as in asking what the past will mean if the future is anticipated in a certain way.

The last chapter considered the dynamics and interpersonal history of ties and traditions as they figure in the meaning of home care. This chapter turns to what commonly is portrayed as the eventual future of increasingly impaired elderly—institutionalization—which usually means nursing home placement.

Time and Personal Adjustment

The phrases "shake the past" or "forget the past" are regularly used as a guide for positive personal adjustment. This is based on the idea that time and experience can be divided into distinct portions, which can be selectively emphasized, suppressed, or eliminated. Given effective management of life history, one can successfully dwell in a particular portion of a lifetime. Commonplace remarks such as "You're living totally in the past" and "You're always thinking about the future" suggest as much.

Intervention conveys preference for living in the present. Tradition is viewed as a likely cause of many troubles in daily life, preventing those affected from casting off troubles linked with past ties and forming relations appropriate to present conditions. By and large, living in the past is a negative adjustment. A caregiver's living in the past suggests a lack of realism about present responsibilities. The care receiver who expects treatment in accordance with past obligations or sentiments places an unrealistic burden on the caregiver. Positive adjustment means being "realistic," which, in turn, means being oriented to present realities. The idea that one might be positively adjusted by placing past obligations to the care receiver at the center of one's current relationship with him or her is unrealistic.

The problem with the future is not that one is likely to "live there," which would be the future equivalent of living in the past, but that one might persist in dwelling on positive times to come. Chance is best figured in terms of present conditions rather than in terms of uncertain future prospects. In other words, the future is best treated as an extension of the present. Given the frailty of care receivers, the aging process, and the increasing burden of care, the future bodes negatively unless it is faced realistically. Present conditions are likely to get worse. For a positive adjustment it is altogether reasonable to raise the question of the care receiver's institutionalization.

A present-centered preference applies to all, not just the caregiver. Ideally, frail elderly are expected in time to make the transition from avoiding the prospect of nursing home placement to the realization that increasing impairment is beyond the capability of the most devoted caregiver. The much used phrase, "the second victim," aptly conveys a negative outcome. Frail elderly who are not lucid enough to take stock of caregiving in support of ostensibly realistic decisions can be spoken for. Statements like "Martha [a demented care receiver] would realize the burden of care if she could and would want you [the caregiver] to think about a nursing home" are commonplace. Even the caregiver can be spoken for. A former caregiver who has placed her husband in a nursing home and is now a facilitator puts it this way in explaining to a caregiving wife what the wife "really" feels despite heroic efforts and claims to the contrary:

Katherine [the caregiver wife], we all know what you're saying. Each of us has been there, believe me. Oh, how we've been there! But have you asked yourself what you're saying? Have you really, really listened to yourself lately? My dear, you sound a lot like I did last year when Bill [her now institutionalized husband] was at home vegetating. He didn't even know my name. I kept saying to myself, "I'm his wife. I love him. I know he'd do the same for me if I was in his shoes." Katherine, face it. You're not that different. Face up to what you're really feeling right now. Forget the past for a minute. I know now that what I was really saying to myself underneath it all was, "Bill, I'm sorry, really sorry, but it's just too much for me now and I need to do something before I fall apart." I just know that's what you're feeling Katherine, but I know, too, how you don't want to admit it.

Of course not all caregivers accept such interpretations of their presumed "real" thoughts and feelings about the past, present, and future. In practice, the question of institutionalization presents caregivers and family members with diverse ways of addressing the future as it weighs on the present.

While sympathy is extended to anyone burdened by caregiving, ideally, in due course the realistic caregiver comes around to display the proper attitude. When the proper attitude is not forthcoming, the caregiver or family member is said to be unrealistic and, in the final analysis, a "martyr" or "denying." The martyr does not accord with the linear view of personal adjustment because he or she is said to "need" to prove that a tradition of filial responsibility is dutifully in effect. The denier does not accord with the linear view because he or she does not realize what really is being felt "underneath it all." The martyr gives priority to tradition while the denier unwittingly ignores the significance of newly emerging ties with the care receiver.

From the nursing home and support groups to family homes, attendant professional workers by and large take formal account of responses to the question of institutionalization in linear terms. Dora's four-stage interpretation of Harry's adjustment to the care of his wife Ruth is exemplary. References are made to both popular and professional literature conveying the same point of view. Professional competence is signaled by references to "models," "theories," and other formal designs claimed to represent the course of personal adjustment in the broader context of the institutionalization decision.

Professional workers can be annoyed by the conceptual obligations of their competence (Gubrium, Buckholdt & Lynott, 1989). For example, a nurse who, despite a professional commitment to represent adjustment in linear terms, pleads with her colleagues to attend to experiential timings, informing them she is aware that there is more to the care experience than a course of adjustment. But, like the past that is said to tell only of things long gone, thereby constituting the realistic present, the linear view is not simply set aside for what is sensed to be more diversely organized. Dissention risks casting doubt on professional competence itself.

The language of stages, adjustment, past abnegation, current reality, and future forecasting based on the present is virtually in the air everyone breathes about the why's and wherefore's of responding to caregiving. In this regard, what the service provider conveys in the capacity of a professional merely reflects what is generally understood (Gubrium, 1986a, 1989a).

"Hard Comes with the Territory": Myra's Story

Myra is a home caregiver and nursing home volunteer. I met her while doing field work in a residential care facility for blind elderly (Gubrium, 1980a, 1980b). Her name regularly comes up in patient care conferences in connection with a patient who, according to the staff, Myra is "very close to and concerned for." The patient, Bill, is an old friend of Myra's blind husband, Ernie, and once lived in Myra's neighborhood.

Bill is 89 years old. In his mid-fifties, he was blinded and disabled in an industrial accident. He has been married to the same woman, Ginny, all his life and, according to Myra, lived happily with Ginny in a small, frame house close to the center of town. After the accident, Ginny took a full-time job and Bill accepted work in a sheltered workshop. At 84, he suffered a stroke that left him partially paralyzed and his speech slurred. The couple attempted to manage on their own. When Ginny became ill two years later, things seemed to fall apart. With both of them ailing and Bill almost helpless, Ginny sought help from a local elderly care outreach program, which eventually led to the suggestion that she seek nursing home placement for her husband. She did, and eight months later Bill was moved into Brawley, one of two local nursing homes for the blind.

In many ways, Myra's home care situation with her 87-year-old, blind husband, Ernie, resembles Ginny's before Bill entered Brawley. Ernie's vision worsened later in life. He is now sightless and housebound. Like Bill, Ernie has slowed considerably and exhibits signs of confusion, possibly dementia. Myra, aged 78, is arthritic, but manages to get about town despite the chronic pain in her back. As Ginny and Bill did, Myra and Ernie live on social security and Ernie's pension. Both wives have had trouble managing their husbands' care at home. The husbands' weight and size have made seemingly simple tasks like bathing and dressing difficult.

After Bill was placed at Brawley, Myra made it her business to take up the cause of the sightless, in particular Bill and Ernie. She became an activity volunteer at Brawley and, by bus, visits the nursing home several times weekly. She alternates between volunteering in the crafts and games area of the activity department and a decided vigilance over Bill's care. Myra's interest in blindness is more than practical; she reads voraciously about it and talks at length with anyone she meets who knows the slightest thing about how the blind think, feel, and manage their lives.

Whenever the staff has questions about Bill's health status or plans for his continuing care, they make a point of seeking Myra's advice. For all practical purposes, Myra is considered to be Bill's family. Ginny rarely visits the nursing home, having become incapacitated herself. She depends on Myra to keep apprised of her husband.

Myra's thoughts on the question of institutionalization are informed by two time tracks. Her approach to Ginny and to Bill's institutionalization is guided by a linear model. Discussing Bill's placement at Brawley, Ginny's response to the institutionalization of her husband, and the couple's current situation, Myra describes three or four stages of personal adjustment. In contrast, Myra's orientation to Ernie's home care is placed distinctly in the context of difficult, but normal family living. In discussing her husband Ernie's impairments and her own responses to his home care, Myra is clearly unlinear.

Myra discusses in detail how her friend Bill's health worsened, how he became more and more burdensome, and the difficult time Ginny had of it. In the process, she virtually names the familiar ingredients of the original care equation—Bill's impairments, Ginny's burden, her stresses and strain, and the decision to place Bill at Brawley. Myra puts herself in Ginny's shoes, as she explains, in order to convey how Ginny must have felt as she witnessed Bill grow feebler and her own capacity to care for him wane.

> You can imagine what she's [Ginny] gone through—the wringer. When I put myself in her shoes . . . maybe I have a bad habit of doing that, putting my nose in places I shouldn't . . . well, I can't help thinking and feeling that you get to a point where you just can't take it anymore. You've seen Bill. He's a very big man and I know I'd have a hard time handling him. I have a hard enough time with my Ernie. Is he ever a bundle! Like I said, you can see what Ginny went through before she finally realized, for her own good really, that something had to be done about it.

The comments and sentiments accord with the ideal personal responses of the caregiver depicted in the linear view of personal adjustment.

As Myra elaborates the story of Bill's institutionalization, she speaks as if one thing realistically led to another. Her comments are very touching, giving the impression that it is Myra herself who has actually gone through Ginny and Bill's leave-taking. At points, it sounds like Myra really is Ginny. Myra seems to say as much as she repeatedly speaks of putting herself in Ginny's shoes. Myra details the "many things Ginny and Bill have been to each other," that the two were best friends from the very beginning, the fear Ginny felt as she became unable to care for her husband, and her final realization that she had to forget all that and think about the future.

> Poor Ginny. They've meant so much to each other; they were the best of friends. They were so close; they were always together. Believe you me, you don't build up that kind of relationship over 50 years and just drop it like a hot potato. When I put myself in her shoes, I know how she feels. I feel it too. You get that kind of emptiness deep down inside. When you even dare to think about him not being around and seeing his face . . . you know, just hearing him breathe next to you . . . you

kinda get scared thinking about how you might have to give him up because neither of you can make it together. The feeling can get to you more than the lifting and all that, worse than the burden. It gets a hold of you and makes you worse than the burden. It gets a hold of you and makes you so, so blue. I think it's thinking about the loss that's the problem. When you think about it too much, it's like you feel yourself dying inside because he's so much a part of you. [Long pause.] A person just can't keep thinking like that. You just can't or you drive yourself crazy. You just have to face up to the fact that you can't handle him anymore and you just have to forget the past, be realistic, and think about what's ahead. Believe you me, knowing Ginny as I do, it was the only thing to do. I would have done the very same thing in her shoes.

When Myra conveys the thoughts and sentiments of her own related experiences with her husband, it is an entirely different story, equally reasonable and heartfelt. Asked if she has not been having the same difficulties with Ernie as Ginny had with Bill and whether there might not be a point when she herself has to think about a nursing home, Myra responds:

Yeah, Ernie's a lot of trouble, but I never, never think of him being a burden. After all, I'm his wife and he's family. Like I say, when it comes to your husband, your wife, your children, whoever, you do just do what you have to do, nothing less. That's the way it was with my parents and that's the way it is with me. Of course, sometimes it's hard; believe me it's very hard sometimes. But isn't life hard all around? Just working for a living is hard! They say raising kids is hard. But you don't give up on them, do you? Hard comes with the territory. That's the story of my life.

Probing further, Myra is asked if what she refers to as "trouble" does not become a personal burden in time and grow to a point where the only reasonable option for the good of all concerned is to end it. Again, Myra refuses to link trouble and burden. Trouble to her is simply part of life, to be accepted and dealt with, not lamented or escaped. Facing up to, and accepting, trouble *is* being realistic. What she has with Ernie is trouble, a great deal of it, which she later describes as making her tired, weary, and admittedly desperate at times. Trouble for Myra is categorically distinct from burden. Burden is what Ginny experienced, for which Myra feels genuinely sorry. As far as Myra is concerned, trouble has little or no

direct bearing on "giving up," which in this case means institutionalization. Only burden suggests it is reasonable to give up, warranted
in Ginny's situation. As far as members of her own family are concerned, Myra holds to a tradition in which burden is unthinkable.

In a certain respect, what Ernie presents to Myra is similar to
what Ruth in the last chapter presents to her husband Harry. The
difference is that Myra takes trouble to be part of the normal expectations of daily living, which in turn is what caring for family is believed
to entail. Harry, in contrast, refuses to link what he calls "tasks" with
his devotion to his wife. Taken together, the two stories show that the
experiential linkages of ties can cast their meaning in diverse ways.
Harry divides his ties with Ruth into two categories: instrumental
and interpersonal. Myra embeds her own ties with her husband, not
Ginny's with Bill, in the framework of normal daily living.

"You Keep Looking Back and Thinking": Ginny's Story

Myra makes it possible to befriend Ginny. It seems from the
many times Myra and I talk of Ginny that Ginny is an old acquaintance. When I meet her, it is evident that she already is acquainted
with me. Myra has told her about my research at the nursing home.
Ginny remarks that it is so nice that I am looking into the way
patients adjust to nursing home life and hopes that her husband in
particular is doing well. She makes a special point of telling me that
Myra is fond of me and that any friend of Myra's is a friend of hers.
It is a propitious beginning.

I am prepared to talk about the experience of institutionalizing a family member. As ethnographic interviews go, our exchanges are to be open-ended, focused on specific topics, and guided
only to the extent that the respondent is encouraged to present the
way he or she sorts and assembles experience. I expect to ask about
her thoughts and feelings as she considered placing Bill in a nursing
home as well as how she responded after the decision was made and
Bill left home. From what I have been repeatedly told by Myra
(speaking for Ginny), Ginny has come around to where she feels
that placing Bill at Brawley was the best thing to do in the circumstance. I plan to organize my inquiry and responses to Ginny's
comments in terms of this course of personal adjustment, asking

questions about her life history with Bill, what life together was like before Bill became an invalid, how she responded to caregiving, and her reactions as she herself grew ill and frail. I expect Ginny to convey a linear version of related experiences. My assumption is that she will look back over her interpersonal history and sort through it in the way Myra presented it to me (Gubrium & Lynott, 1983).

Surpisingly, as I speak with Ginny, it is apparent that the past, present, and future have a different organization. Not only do I learn that a course of personal adjustment is something one can go through repeatedly, but that its implicit linearity can be recurrently reevaluated for whether it is, as Ginny puts it, "really the right way to think about all of this." In other words, not only does Ginny experience several courses of personal adjustment, but she theorizes about it in the process!

Asked to tell what went through her mind when she considered Bill's continued home care, Ginny talks about the past, her thoughts, and her feelings. It is soon evident that, to Ginny, the past cannot be separated from her present attempt to get a handle on it. In a lengthy commentary, she remarks:

> Look, young man, don't take this the wrong way, but I don't think you ever, ever really know what you felt. At that time, I was convinced, I guess, that it was the right thing to do [place Bill in a nursing home]. Anyway, I kept telling myself that. They say that you go through this kind of thing . . . you know, you don't want to do it, you don't even want to think about it. They say you're denying . . . I think that's what the social worker said. I can't remember that much now. Anyway, that stuff does goes through your mind. But, you know, Jay, thinking back, you just don't know what it was. Was I trying to keep from facing up to all the work and all the bother that Bill was then? After all, he was my husband! We were very close, really best friends. I was always thinking of him. I guess. But now that you ask . . . and I've asked myself this over and over . . . what went through my mind [long pause] You keep looking back and thinking. I wish I knew.

There are points in our discussion when it seems that both of us, right then, are composing Ginny's past as we move along. It occurs to me that, from the point of view of a "hard science" methodology, I might be contributing to the production of data and not being neutral in gathering the facts of Ginny's testimony. At the same time, in her own way, Ginny keeps telling me that each of her own reflections on what happened has been doing the same thing. She seems to think that this is natural (Rubinstein, 1989b). Indeed, at one point, she validates this process of data production by remarking in passing that it isn't natural not to have "second thoughts about your life," "take stock of what you felt," and "try to make some sense of things."

> *They say . . . Myra keeps saying this, too . . . maybe she just wants me to feel better. They say that you have to bury the past, the past is the past, and you have to start to think about the future. Even my neighbor says that you can't live in the past. Well . . . I'm not such a boob. What future? You do have a past. Can I deny that I had a husband? You tell me this. Can I say that? Can I forget that he's not with me here now and every night he's not here? Can I? Sure, you have second thoughts about your life. Who doesn't? It's a natural thing to do. You take stock of what you felt and try to make sense of things. When you get to be my age [79 years old] and you're home alone like this, that's all you have. Did you ever think about that? Should I give that up, too? It's natural; it's part of you. Yeah, it's very sad to think about what had to happen. . . . Go ahead, ask more questions.*

As the conversation unfolds, at times we are talking about a linear model of personal adjustment without actually naming it. Ginny refers to how one in general adjusts to "these things," what "they say" one goes through, and in the process raises pointed questions about whether what "they say" is really how one "goes through" it. She describes how she used to think about what she was feeling and compares it to what she now believes one goes through. The story repeatedly challenges a linear view of personal adjustment. In saying "You keep looking back," she tells me that the past is inevitably tied to the present and future, and that to assemble and reassemble it in some reasonable fashion is part of life. Without this there would not be much left.

Looking back, Ginny agonizingly wonders if it is really right to forget. There is a definite moral undertone to her theoretical musings. She contemplates whether in having foreseen a future overburdened with Bill's care and suffering and then trying to forget the past, she has been selfish, thinking only of her own comfort. There are points when the past itself seems to represent Bill, and the present and future to represent Ginny. Can it be, she asks, that her effort to tear the past away from the present and future, means that she has decided to tear Bill from her life? She is angry that time—which "they say" passes—has been allowed to take control of her thoughts, and she now feels guilty about seeing things so simply. She is annoyed that her adjustment is the thing she let be the focus of her response to the situation, surmising that this is the ultimate self-indulgence.

Informing me that Myra, in her kindly way, at first kept telling her not to punish herself, Ginny indicates that it is not punishment that she is now inflicting on herself, but rather an attempt to sort through what has happened. As Ginny repeats, "It's something you just have to do." In a bit of dark humor, she states:

> *Maybe I should be like some of those in the nursing home. Huh? They can't remember a thing. That would be a stroke of good luck, wouldn't it? They're happy as a lark. [Pauses and looks straight at me.] Yeah, and I know what you're going to say, too. They have no mind either. So what! [She snickers.]*

This story is not about one who has more or less gone through stages of personal adjustment to loss "for her own good," as Myra has put it. While some might see her as stuck at a stage short of complete resolution, it is evident that Ginny has thought at length about, and continued to ponder the meaning of, stages, adjustment, and resolution. If anything is a theme of her story, it is the bearing of the idea of personal adjustment on the interpersonal experience of the past, present, and future. The question that does not seem to go away is whether adjustment means that when one breaks a tie, one severs oneself from its related past to show that one cared more about oneself than another. It is no wonder that Ginny "takes the bad with the good," as she likes to put it, keeping alive the full memory of Bill's life with her over the years despite the painful associated feelings.

For better or worse, this caregiver continues to actively give shape and content to what happened in the past. As we talk, she comments on how one sees events in so many different ways and experiences so many different feelings in "thinking about things." In the time I spend with her, I find that reflection itself shapes adjustment.

Companionship: Lucy's Story

Lucy's story provides an added dimension, showing how issues of companionship and possible isolation intrude on the question of institutionalization. From Lucy's perspective, her caregiving experience with her husband, Melvin, is a narrative of time well spent, with someone and not alone. The story highlights a tie Ginny looks back on with both regret and desire.

Lucy is an active member of a local chapter of the Alzheimer's Disease and Related Disorders Association (ADRDA). She helped to organize it and its support group for family caregivers. At its founding, she had already been caring for her wheelchair-bound husband at home for several years.

Lucy is 71 and Melvin 77. Earlier in life, Mel was involved in union activities and local politics. He had even unsuccessfully run for mayor. Lucy had had a life filled with volunteer work and advocacy. What originally attracted her to Mel was that "he was so interesting, active, and intelligent," as she explains. Just as Lucy herself supported myriad causes and held strong opinions about a number of others, Mel made causes a major purpose of his life. Lucy's connection with the ADRDA was one more spoke in a wheel of lifelong social concern. According to Lucy, despite their age, both continue to be outspoken critics of injustice and inequality. The indirect benefit of this activity is not just political satisfaction. As Lucy explains, "It's what keeps your head clear and your heart strong."

While Mel has been tentatively diagnosed as having Alzheimer's, Lucy is skeptical. She figures that Mel is just too alert for that, even though his mind occasionally wanders and he does get things confused. In any case, it is not the confusion that poses the greatest time commitment for her, but Mel's physical cares, in particular his frequent incontinence, immobility, and arthritic backpain. But as in Harry's story in the last chapter and in Myra's in this one, these are, to Lucy, part of the inexorable travails of life.

This is not to say that what these caregivers face, day in and day out, is trivial, nor that their responses are limited to the giving of care and personal musings on it. In her support group, Lucy, for one, regularly lectures for others' benefit about the impact on the caregiver of giving care, especially for the Alzheimer's disease patient. She also makes it her business to call on those who are desperate, offering comfort and advice. She shares with other care-givers the knowledge and skill she has accumulated in Mel's home care. She contributes to her ADRDA chapter newsletter for caregivers. She helps to organize local public service programs dealing with caregiving, making a veritable mission of spreading the word of the "36-hour day" that home care entails. Her home and caregiving experience have been featured in a chapter-sponsored videotape.

The heart of her tie with Melvin, however, is far from such matters. Foremost, Mel is Lucy's daily companion—a friend. Despite his confusion, and because they have the same interests and commitments, Mel is her "partner in crime," as she likes to put it. Lucy is known for her keen sense of humor, which comes through in response to a support group discussion concerning the question of when "it's time," that is, time to consider nursing home placement:

> *Like Rhonda [another caregiver] says, well, "Mel's my main man." He's my partner in crime. He's always making me laugh, even when he does crazy things, like when he tried to dress himself and he got my panties out of the drawer and tried to put them on. You should have seen him! The old union man with ladies' panties around his ankles. [Details her response.] How could I think about putting this guy in a nursing home? What would I do without him? He's the closest friend I have.*

Lucy's view of the companionship Mel provides does not go unchallenged. Support group participants are well acquainted with the "denial" that caregivers can present in the course of responding to impairment and strain. It is a language the facilitator frequently uses and a commonplace topic in the popular literature participants read. Some consider Lucy to be denying the inevitable, that is, the prospect of Mel's continual decline and eventual need for professional care. Participants know, too, that some caregivers become "martyrs" in home care and consider Lucy, especially, to have this tendency.

Lucy is aware of the accusations, but discounts them. In a conversation I have with her in her home, she takes account of them in terms of what she calls "the positive side."

> *Some of them can't see anything but the downside of things. Sometimes that's all they can say. They're stressed out, they say. They can't take it. Any time you say that there's any good about it, they jump all over you.*

[Pause.] Of course, they're not all like that. But there's a positive side. But it [the criticism] can get to you. [Elaborates her response to the criticism.] Sure it's hard. I won't deny it. But Mel's such a cutup. He makes me laugh all the time. Sure, sometimes he doesn't know it's me in the house; he thinks I'm a strange woman. Get that! A strange woman. He could be so lucky. But [pause] it's someone in the house. It's someone to talk to. Mel's always there. I have my man around me all the time, as confused as he is.

I ask her whether there would not be a time when she, indeed, would have to consider looking into the possibility of a nursing home and whether it is perhaps the cost of institutionalization that prevents her from doing anything about it. Again the companionship theme comes forth:

Time? Well . . . his time's my time. Time, you say? No. We're close friends, Mel and me. I'd say we just pass the time, like two lovebirds. . . . The cost. Well, the cost is high, yes, but really we can afford it. I can afford to have someone come in here, too, and help me out. But why should I? It's not the cost. Well . . . yes, for some of them, it's the cost. Even for them it's not only that [cost]. After all, it's a life. It's sad that a government that's supposed to be for the people makes it so hard to grow old. It's very hard to be old in this country.

No, Mel's here to stay . . . with me. Just look at him over there. [Mel's asleep in his wheelchair.] He's no angel, but he's all I have. He keeps me company. We've got those birds and this old mutt here, but they can't replace him. Sometimes he's so confused that it comes out jibberish. But I help him out and, well, if you're patient, you know what he wants. I say things for him sometimes and he nods yes or no, if he can. That's what we do, Mel and me. And, boy, he'll come out with the craziest things sometimes. I'll be laughing for days just thinking about it. Maybe I'm a martyr, but he's the only friend I've got.

I couldn't imagine me living in this house alone. Who would I talk to? The dog? People would think I was crazy. I'd think I was crazy! . . . Loneliness. Being alone when you're old. To me, that's the worst. [Elaborates.] No thanks. I'll take Mel whatever way he comes. [She approaches Mel and caresses him.] You wouldn't know it from seeing him like this, but there's a lot to this guy.

To Never Be a Burden: Dan's Story

Perusing the literature on the dynamics of caregiving for the elderly, one would think the sole voice in the process was the caregiver's. If others' experiences are heard, it is family members'. Rarely do we hear the voice of the care receiver. He or she remains in the background, as if all that mattered were the impairment presented to the caregiver and the resulting response.

Yet as we saw in the last chapter, despite Ruth's being relatively incommunicative, Harry took bits and pieces of her demeanor as signs of her enduring desires. We saw, too, how Sally's past relationship with her mother continued to intrude into their current affairs, as if the mother were now lucidly present in her life. In this chapter, Mel's companionship offers daily rounds of humor, conversation, and good cheer in addition to trials and tribulations. Still, none of these stories presented the care receiver as explicitly involved in decision making concerning institutionalization.

There are stories of care receivers who do directly participate. Dan's is one. He is 73 years old, has suffered a paralyzing stroke, is confined to a wheelchair, and has emphysema associated with a lifetime of heavy smoking. His wife died in an automobile accident when she was 57. Dan has never remarried and continues to mourn for his wife. While he is admittedly forgetful at times, he claims to be as alert as the best of them. Until his stroke, he managed the family home and kept two dogs and a cat, although the emphysema made him weak. After his stroke, things became much more difficult for him.

I became acquainted with Dan in connection with a field study of images of care and recovery in a rehabilitation hospital (Gubrium & Buckholdt, 1982). Following his stroke, he was hospitalized for physical therapy. His three children and several of his adult grandchildren dutifully participated in the hospital's family conferences, stroke program, and support group for family members. Since rehabilitation patients, especially those with some permanent paralysis, commonly leave the hospital less capable than they were before the accidents that caused their disabilities, a common question in discharge planning is whether the patient will return home. A related question is whether institutional placement or extended care is in order. It is through my hospital contacts with the family and later follow-up of the case that I learned how complex the part of the care receiver can be in addressing the question.

By his own account, Dan has always been the kind of person who does not want to be a burden on anyone, especially his family. According to Dan's three children, even before the stroke, Dan regularly told them that he didn't ever want to be a burden on them. It is a sentiment that I heard Dan repeat many times over the course of his hospitalization. One time, in a long and rather difficult conversation with him in the lounge area outside his room, Dan remarked:

> *I'm very proud of them three; they're my life. When Milly [his wife] passed . . . it was very sudden and very sad . . . I told them that I didn't ever want them to think that they had to take care of their old man. [Elaborates.] Oh, I took care of things, but it wasn't the same without her around the place. After I started to get this emphysema thing and it got worse . . . and then this stroke that gave me this bum arm and . . . it's hard to talk . . . [long pause]. Well, it isn't the same. But it's my problem and those kids of mine, they got a life of their own. Like I told you, I'm not going to be a burden on anyone.*

Dan believes that parents have an obligation to raise their children to the best of their ability. Children need to be loved and made to feel secure, he frequently points out. That much he feels he and Milly have accomplished, even while it was done in the style they had hoped. Dan also believes that parents should never, in turn, expect their children to care for them. Children and grandchildren have a "lifetime of living to do," Dan says, and the older generation has no business making claims on the young when the aged grow frail. He informs me that he has made plans to sell his house and has decided to move to a nearby, "very nice" nursing home where he knows a few residents.

One complication in the matter is that Dan suspects that his three children feel differently about this decision. He asks me several times how I would handle the situation, in particular how to insist on making arrangements for his own institutional care following discharge from the hospital and not hurt the children's feelings. Dan does not want to seem ungrateful to them for all the love and care they have given him. He does not want to give the impression that he is finished with them. Sighing, he states, "It really gets to me when Karen [his oldest daughter] asks me, 'Daddy, don't you think we love you and want you to come home with us?'"

The family has a strong tradition of mutual help. As long as Dan is relatively fit to care for himself at home, family ties are strengthened each time Dan helps the children and grandchildren, and they in turn help Dan. After Dan suffers a stroke and is weakened by emphysema, the tradition of mutual help, as always, comes into play. The three children expect to care for their father in their own homes after his discharge from the hospital.

At the same time, Dan's firm belief about the younger generation's not owing anything to the older lurks in the background. Well aware of this, the children ask members of Dan's treatment team and fellow participants of a support group for families of stroke patients to "get him to see things our way," as they put it. While they want to please their father, they are, at the same time, fully committed to caring for him on their own.

In espousing his philosophy of elderly self-care, Dan remarks several times that he has made sure that, whatever comes, he will be able to take care of himself in his old age and never be a burden to his children. When I raise the question of the cost of nursing home care with the children, they share the opinion that there are many important things to think about in making such a decision and that cost is the least of them.

It is not altogether clear how the question of Dan's discharge destination is resolved. Eventually, Dan is discharged to his son's home. It is agreed that Dan will rotate living with the children. In retrospect, Dan reports that things seemed to just happen the way they did and that, at the time, he did not have the energy to make much fuss about it. The children explain that they had been convinced by experiences shared in the hospital's support group that things have a way of working themselves out in close-knit families. The social worker recalls that she advised they try home care for a while before deciding on an alternative.

In the months following discharge, it is evident that there is more to the meaning of "things working out" than established accommodations of daily living. The residential arrangement goes as smoothly as expected. Dan spends approximately six months in each child's home. Yet, there is a virtually unmentionable strain between the children and their father. No one seems able to resolve it, or even to talk about it. Everything has worked out nicely except for the silent awareness that Dan does not want to be kept by his children because, to him, it means being burdensome.

The children remind me that none of them has ever felt burdened. Their father's feelings trouble them. Len, the son, remarks, "I just sense that Daddy isn't happy living with us and it really makes us all feel very sad that we can't take care of him and keep him a part of the family." When I talk to Dan in private, he mentions that the children are most accommodating, but, at the same time, suspects they think he is uncomfortable depending on them, repeating that he does not want them to think him ungrateful. Dan also feels "ashamed," as he mentions, about having to intrude on the domestic affairs of their "happy little homes." The situation resembles the quiet desperation of what Glaser and Strauss (1965) call a context of "mutual pretense."

Neither Dan as care receiver nor the children as caregivers play minor parts in the story. If anything, it is Dan, the care receiver, who is most concerned with the burden of care. When push comes to shove, which Dan asserts is "just a matter of time," it is his intention to quickly resolve the home care situation by insisting on being moved into a nursing home. The daily burdens of care are bad enough; the family's tradition of responsibility and Dan's exception to it in his case make matters worse.

A "Woman in the Middle" Imagines Placement: Mary's Story

Mary is the 62-year-old caregiver of her mother, Nina, who is 84 and suffers from Alzheimer's disease. They live across the street from each other in separate houses. After Nina's husband dies, younger members of the extended family move in with Nina at various times. It offers a modicum of independence from parents for the young people and provides live-in supervision for Nina. Mary is the primary caregiver.

Mary always has lived near her mother, either in the same neighborhood, in each other's homes, or, currently, on the same street. They have been best friends. As Mary remarks, "When Mother was up and about, people used to think we were older and younger sisters; we were always together." Nina's forgetfulness, confusion, and occasional incontinence cause Mary as much emotional distress as it is physically burdensome. Mary misses the "old Nina," the company they kept, and the bosom companionship they provided each other.

Mary's husband, Don, always has been cool to Nina. As Nina's dementia, physical health, and her presence in and about his home increasingly takes Mary away from him and the family, Don's resentment flares. But Mary understands:

> *Poor Don. I know what he's going through. Who wouldn't? I'm torn between having to tend to Mother and keeping him company. A man needs a wife around. It's his companion. Still, she's my mother and I really, really feel that, as long as she's with us [Mary knocks on wood], I'll try to make her life as comfortable as possible. [Details her daily cares for Nina.]*

> *Mother and I were always very, very close. I think you'd say we were best friends. Don was pretty good about it, but I think underneath he really resented it, especially when I took time away from him and the boys [their three children]. In a way, I was lucky to have boys, because the men in the family did a lot of men things together anyway. I always wished I had had a daughter though, like Mother.*

Judged by the literature on social support, home care, and institutionalization, Nina's situation gets high marks for keeping her in the community and out of a nursing home (Johnson & Grant, 1985, chap. 4). A major factor in institutionalization is the lack of a support system. In Nina's case, various adult grandchildren reside with her offering supervision and a daughter is conveniently available for personal cares and home management. But Nina's home care is not only affected by a support system. A wider social network of ties indirectly impinges on the support system.

While a social network is a configuration of ties, it is not necessarily supportive. As Morgan (1989) points out in a study of adjustment to widowhood, social networks do not always "really make it easier." The implication is that the broader network of social ties should be paid closer attention in examining the effect of social support on the chance of institutionalization. On balance, part of a network of social ties actually may "push" a care receiver out of the home while another part may only weakly "pull" the receiver back in (Gubrium & Lynott, 1987).

In Mary's story, Don is exasperated with what he sees as his wife's and children's unrealistic devotion. It requires unacceptable time commitments. To complicate matters, Mary's active participation in a local support group for caregivers of Alzheimer's disease victims conveys mixed messages about whether the time for nursing home placement is rapidly approaching in Nina's case. Certain support group friends suggest that it is unrealistic for Mary to continue carrying the daily load of her mother's care, while others feel differently.

Nina's support system is virtually under siege as members of her broader social network variously perceive looming troubles, not mere inconveniences, in the home care situation. Mary has become the proverbial "woman in the middle," caught between the claims and commitments of separate generations and the contrasting sentiments of respected friends and acquaintances (Brody, 1981). In this context, the question of whether "it's time" is not simple and straightforward. The many versions of her story confuse Mary: what she has always told herself, what her husband is now vociferously demanding, and what others variously convey.

Mary's story also shows that the question of institutionalization is as much imaginatively addressed as it is figured in relation to versions of particular concrete conditions of care. Mary contemplates "both sides"—what it would mean for both her and her mother if Nina were placed in a nursing home and what it would mean for them if Nina remained at home in Mary's care. In a related conversation in her home, Mary talks about the dilemma. She starts by poignantly reminding me of what she knows we both have heard, time and again, concerning how one placed in a nursing home "must feel" leaving a home and lifelong ties behind to spend his or her remaining days alone in an institution.

> *You can imagine how it must feel to leave your family behind—all your friends, your kids, your home, all of it. Think about it. It's done. It's over. There you are, all alone, nothing of yours around to remind you that you're Jay or you're Mary. It must be awful. That's what I think of, day in and day out, when I think about what Don and the others say I should do. I know they mean well . . . and poor Don . . . what am I going to do with him? He's suffering too.*

I remind Mary that we both also have heard caregivers say that there gets to be a point when "it's time," when the Alzheimer's disease patient does not recognize the caregiver any more, or even those known a lifetime. When I mention that perhaps such persons would not suffer so, Mary sharpens the image presented earlier:

Yes. I know. But did you ever stop to think, like I have, that maybe . . . I know she [Nina] sounds very confused and she can't tell us much. . . . Maybe deep, deep down inside, maybe she knows what's going on, like she's trying to reach out but isn't able to say it so it comes out right? Who really knows? I thought about that real hard when Cathy [a support group participant] . . . that poor woman. I really feel sorry for her. Since she put Hal [Cathy's husband] at Millhaven [a nursing home], she just cries and cries every time she thinks about how he feels in there. I think about it . . . Mother in there and she's in a wheelchair, and like she calls out something nobody can understand and what she wants to say is like "Mary, Mary, please help me. Mary, come and get me. Mary, hug me because I'm so alone." [Long pause.] Everyone has a soul, you know. We can't just forget that. [Mary weeps.]

Mary of course knows that there is another version to the story. She hears it told in varied detail in her support group. It is a story of a caregiver who cannot admit, despite all evidence to the contrary, that a loved one has, for all practical purposes, died as a person. Mary has heard others describe how the Alzheimer's patient, in time, becomes an "empty shell" and how life for those who insist on caring for such an individual is like a "funeral that never ends." Mary knows, too, that this story has holes. As she asks implicitly in the preceding extract, is that so-called empty shell really empty? How can one know for sure? Maybe Alzheimer's is an incapacity to communicate, not the death of a soul. What is known of such matters in the final analysis (Gubrium, 1986b, 1988c)?

Mary says that there are times she believes what the evidence suggests, which is that Nina is no longer that mother Mary once knew. On these occasions, Mary wants to believe that Don, her husband, is right. She wishes desperately to be rid of her alleged denial. As she has so often been told, she wants to put the past behind, look to the future, and begin to think about her own health and well-being. She hopes to be on her way to making the "right decision." Yet a particularly telling comment of hers suggests that the process of adjustment is more an idea she has to convince herself of than it represents what caregivers actually go through: "Maybe if I keep telling myself that that's the way it is [the various stages one goes through], I'll eventually believe it and things'll work out like they say they should." Again we find that linear time and personal adjustment are as much themes applied to experience as they are facts of caregiving.

Implications for the Professional Caregiver

Consider adjustment and adaptation as contrasting terms for designating implications for intervention.

ADJUSTMENT VERSUS ADAPTATION

The language of adjustment suggests there is a standard of conduct around which to organize attitudes and behaviors in response to life events. Success, as in successful adjustment, is measured by the standard. When one conforms to the standard, he or she is said to be adjusted, a positive outcome. When the subject does not conform, there is maladjustment, a negative outcome. It is a rather restrictive approach to the relation between life events and personal change.

According to the linear view, to adjust to the burden of care means that, preferably sooner than later, one follows stages of change in psychosocial orientation to the care receiver, from concern with cure and progress to an emphasis on personal well-being and overall family welfare. When this does not occur in a relatively expeditious manner, the caregiver is said to be "unrealistic," "a martyr," or "denying," among other terms of reference for negative outcomes.

The language of adaptation is less restrictive. It implies a more active caregiver. He or she is viewed as capable of designing and assembling diverse understandings of the caregiving experience, not necessarily drawing inspiration from the idea of a unidirectional chain of events and responses, that is, from impairment, burden, stress, and strain to institutionalization. While a particular caregiver, in fact, may organize his or her experience according to a linear vision of adjustment, from the point of view of adaptation, it is only one way of responding to the care experience. Other patterns of adaptation exist as possible solutions.

LANGUAGE, TIMING, AND INTERVENTION

The languages reflect more than stylistic preferences. They actually instruct one's approach to clients and guide interventions, encouraging contrasting orientations to psychosocial timing. In the language of adjustment, the future is fixed in principle, that is, the family caregiver follows along specified stages of change and adjusts or does not, as the case may be. Clock time dominates experience. In a manner of speaking, in time "it's time" to consider the question of institutionalization, in time the frail elder is placed in a nursing home for the good of all concerned, in time the caregiver resumes a positive attitude, and so on. The professional worker who orients to adjustment as *the* way to think about the care experience harbors a kind of fatalism in dealing with the client, closing off invented options. In contrast, in the language of adaptation, the future is yet to come. Timing has an open horizon. The caregiver is given rein to make the best of what he or she can manage and affectively afford.

The stories presented in this chapter suggest that it is important to keep alert to the distinction between clock time and experiential time. While it was noted at the start that clock time flows forward, the stories show that the future is closely tied to the past. As Mary's story indicates, imagined futures have a way of reversing clock time so that what is contemplated itself shapes the course of change. In the real world, even time is something shaped and assigned meaning, not merely a fixed chronology within whose borders persons adjust (Gubrium & Buckholdt, 1977).

The different languages also tell professional workers whether their interventions are effective. The client who fails to follow a normal course of change not only signals maladjustment, but the possible ineffectiveness of a service provider who has failed to keep the client on track. In the broader context of adaptation, ineffectiveness is not just the result of maladjustment or professional ineffectiveness, but equally the product of how success is defined in the first place. In this context, professional workers fail as much because they are evaluated or evaluate themselves in certain "terms," such as in terms of the facilitation of adjustment.

A language of adaptation permits the professional to entertain recovery and "wellness" in a variety of ways. It diversifies the criteria of professional effectiveness. As the real world's mosaic of care shows, there are many channels for assembling the meaning of troubles, as wide-ranging as their different ties and traditions.

As the linear orientation grows in popularity, becoming professionally prevalent, options for understanding the meaning of the care experience are reduced. The linear model, of course, is only one way of viewing responses to the care experience. But its themes and interpreted experiences have become widespread and stands to be construed as the only way. The stories of this chapter suggest otherwise.

CHAPTER 5

Institutional Living

Erving Goffman (1961b) describes the experience of being institutionalized as a moral career. The term "moral" is a framework of imagery calling attention to the self. He argues that the self is framed in relation to the agendas and categories encountered in the process of institutionalization. The term "career" centers the analysis where the person and the organization intersect, allowing Goffman to trace how institutional processing regulates self-identity. His portrait of the moral career of the mental patient is a study of the first two of three phases—prepatient, inpatient, and expatient. He summarizes the shift from prepatient differences in self-definition to the inpatient homogenization of the self in this way:

> The moral career of a person of a given social category involves a standard sequence of changes in his way of conceiving of selves, including, importantly, his own. These half-buried lines of development can be followed by studying his moral experiences—that is, happenings which mark a turning point in the way in which the person views the world—although the particularities of his view may be difficult to establish (p. 168).

A Local Culture of Opposed Understandings

The approach has a resemblance to the linear model of adjustment. While the linear model applies mainly to the caregiver and the concept of a moral career to the care receiver, both nonetheless view transformations in the self as occurring in phases, stages, and turning points. While, as Goffman states, "the particularities . . . may be difficult to establish," the overall process is a standard sequence. Another similarity is that change goes from bad to worse before it gets better. Upon institutionalization, the mental patient experiences moral degradation. Likewise, with the increasing burden of care, the caregiver experiences stress and strain.

The stories in this chapter offer a different view. Goffman takes the moral themes of the mental hospital to be standard: self-mortification and resocialization. The stories show that the moral themes of the nursing home patient's or resident's adaptation are less uniform. The themes cohere around two sets of opposed understandings concerning the meaning of institutional living. One set is the conflict between an understanding of the nursing facility as a home, on the one side, and as a hospital on the other. Shield's (1988) recent ethnography of daily life in an American nursing home takes this set, so-called conflicting world views, as a framework. The domestic meaning of institutionalization has been similarly approached (Gubrium, 1989a). A second set of opposed understandings is the conflict between the local, present-oriented timing of the nursing home's organizational rhythms and the past/present/future horizon of patients' and residents' life histories. Troubles can be understood in terms of clashes between the opposed ties linked with the timings (Gubrium, 1975).

The sets of understanding are part of the nursing home's local culture and provide the moral context for assigning meaning to one's story in a facility. Institutional living is not simply a matter of adjusting to phases of a moral career defined in standard, linear terms, but rather is a complex process of differentially "touching base," as it were, with opposing senses of what institutional living is all about.

HOME VERSUS HOSPITAL

If one turns to ads for nursing homes in the telephone yellow pages, one is likely to find them described as having homelike atmospheres. The message is that, despite being an institution, the nursing home can provide domestic tranquility, a home away from home for a loved one. For example, the Milwaukee, Wisconsin consumer Yellow Pages (1986-87) state that in the nursing home one can "discover a pleasant home-like environment" (p. 1013), a nursing home can be "truly a place to live—not just to stay" (p. 1015), where one can live "with dignity and respect" in the "safety and security [of] a warm colonial setting" (p. 1015). In the Jacksonville, Florida Yellow Pages (1987–88), it is noted that the nursing home offers both a homelike atmosphere and the benefit of expeditious hospital care, namely, "the efficiency of a hospital, the serenity of a home" (p. 660). The Tampa, Florida, Yellow Pages (1988) embellish the image: "A caring staff will tend to our residents' every need in a home-like setting" (p. 1310).

   The last ad presents members of the "home-like setting" as anything but staff-like and evidently like a caring family. The message here is that institutional living is not only a matter of trading one home for another, but that an institution, like the family, can provide tender, loving care. Thus the ads in the Tampa Yellow Pages point out that "caring is our business" (p. 1310), the Milwaukee consumer Yellow Pages mention that in a nursing home one can "enjoy life in a warm and caring community" (p. 1013), and a Jacksonville counterpart simply states "we care" (p. 659). The terminology is consistent—home, care, warmth, family, security. It is a configuration of concern that presents the opposite of the public view of institutional life as cold, rational, and regulated (Gubrium & Holstein, 1990).

   Shield (1988) suggests that the most important contrasting themes of home versus hospital as a set of opposed understandings are between what she calls "life" and "quality of life." At home, one lives one's life. As the nursing home emulates the hospital's quality of care standards, quality of life is defined according to staffing characteristics, skills, medical records, and other standard items of inspection. A second pair of contrasting themes is spatial and captured in the distinction between residence and room. Contrast centers on the tension between the demand for personal space and privacy on the one hand and the administrative requirements of room assignment and room management on the other. A third pair of opposing themes is the image of staff as employees versus the staff as friends or "family." Shield's fourth pair of opposing themes comes in the differences between rehabilitation and custody, the one aiming for recovery and the other offering maintenance or, as some bluntly say, a final resting place.

In contrast to the developmental logic of a moral career, local cultures of opposed understanding show nursing home life being played out according to dynamic tensions, which are anything but simply linear. At times and under certain conditions, the nursing home is a home. For Phoebe and her clique, their end of the hallway can be quite "cozy," what with its private rooms, warm and solicitous atmosphere, sense of collective security, and local common grounds like "their" bathroom and "their" dayroom. When John ostensibly "invades" the territory and validates the public character of the bathroom, the home becomes the institution no clique member desires, where, if one is not careful, all manner of "riffraff can drift through the place," as Phoebe complains. John's fondness for Miss Hanson, expressed in a tradition of conviviality and banter, is placed in jeopardy as Hanson feels obligated to do her job, that is, be an employee as opposed to John's friend.

On occasion, the opposed understandings of home versus hospital are stretched into extremes. Rather than "caring [being] our business," caring is perceived as punishment. In the end, the hospital-like nursing home is represented as a prison. As Sophie's story in this chapter shows, the prison is an extreme version of what the home ideally is not. Indeed, in some of the field settings, the analogy of the concentration camp is used to convey a sense of institutional confinement.

Life in the nursing home, of course, is not definitely either home-like or hospital-like, nor does it necessarily resemble imprisonment. Rather, local cultural understandings are differentially *used* to organize the meaning of institutional living and convey a sense of what it is like to leave a home. One's sense of self can shift from being defined in terms of family membership to being framed in terms of being hostage, like an inmate, or being in solitary confinement. Just as Edward Said (1978) has shown that the "Orient" has been historically portrayed in terms opposite to what the Occident has taken itself to be, so patients, residents, staff members, and families—even advertisements—use pertinent contrasting themes and opposed understandings to convey their identities and the meaning of institutionalization.

ORGANIZATIONAL TIME VERSUS LIFE HISTORY

Stories suggest that the therapeutic strategy of forgetting the past is a mixed blessing. While a tradition of filial responsibility and an interpersonal history of love and commitment might be viewed as forestalling institutionalization, it also is believed that forgetting the past offers a more realistic attitude in current dire circumstances. Forgetting the past as a basis for making realistic caregiving decisions risks leaving behind a significant part of oneself—what one has meant to another, now means, and will mean in the future. Interpersonal meanings cannot easily be aligned in accordance with the current failures and successes of life. As Ginny remarks in the last chapter, "They say that you have to bury the past. . . . But you do have a past. Can I deny that I had a husband? You tell me this." The meaning of one's life at any point in it, it seems, cannot automatically be confined to the conditions and events of the moment, which, as Ginny suggests, is to risk throwing out everything.

Temporality is the basis for another set of opposed understandings in the nursing home. Organizational rhythms contrast with the personal timings of individual life histories. Institutional living has its distinct way of shaping the relationship between a resident's present, past, and future. The homogenizing tendencies of institutional living—the common daily schedule, the uniform identification of occupants as residents or patients, the rationalization of care and custody—highlight present conditions at the expense of varied individual pasts and futures. Indeed, personal diversity stands to confound organizational rhythms as, say, exceptions to rules of conduct and association are made because of what individual patients have always done or expect to do in the days ahead. Organizational rhythms work to replace individual pasts with patient or resident pasts, framing the future in the same fashion. There is a tendency to dissolve life history into organizational timing and functioning, identity and personhood into organizational roles, statuses, and processing. The personal past and future not only are lost, but biography as well, whose story otherwise stretches into a lifetime.

In the real world, however, the process of institutionalization and the practice of institutional living are not simply (linear) moral careers of self displacement. Like Shield's (1988) conflicting world views of home versus hospital, organizational timing and life history engage lives as a set of practical options for living. Stories reflect diverse encounters with, and articulations of, the opposed understandings. Ties, traditions, and troubles are not only played out in relation to the local tensions of home versus hospital, but equally subject to the opposition of organizational timing and life history. As an organization, the nursing home puts pressure on long-term ties, emphasizing organizational linkages over interpersonal tradition. As staff aim to do jobs uncomplicated by individual pasts and preferences, patients and residents contend with the loss of contact with, and immediate validation of, individual desires and life histories. The particularizing tendencies of life history sustain traditional ties, but they do so against the rationalization of organizational rhythms.

While there are stories of institutionalization and institutional living whose plots feature self transformations designed in Goffmanesque terms, other stories articulate opposed understandings differently. In this regard institutional living, too, features a mosaic of care.

The Occasional Pain of Longing for Home: Sophie's Story

Sophie Bellman believes her family "did right" in placing her at Northwoods, the nursing home where she now resides. Sophie says that she understands how her multiple incapacities make it next to impossible for her working daughter to care for her at home. But Sophie also feels abandoned. She bemoans the fact that her daughter and her son can no longer care for her, like she is a "stranger," a favorite analogy of Sophie's. Sophie categorically distinguishes her life in the nursing home as a patient from her life in the home as a lonely family member. The separate ties form two versions of her story, forming a complex array of opinions and sentiments about institutional living.

As Sophie tells it, after she turned 70, it seemed "all hell broke loose" as misfortune struck. Until then, she could get around "like the best of them." Soon after her birthday, she slipped on the icy sidewalk outside her home and broke her hip. She had been cautioned about venturing outdoors in inclement weather. She knew from many of her friends that broken hips are a common occurrence among older people. But she also knew that broken hips can be survived, as many of her friends mended satisfactorily and quickly. It was Sophie's bad fortune to be different. Following the fall and surgery, she had a difficult recovery. There were complications: repeated infections, pain, depression, and difficulty getting about.

A year later, Sophie still cannot ambulate without the assistance of a walker. She weakens from lack of exercise and extra weight, although she never has been slim. Her legs have a tendency to swell, for which she is given medication. She eventually is confined to a wheelchair. She develops pneumonia and, as she complains, never seems to recover from that either. Her house is burglarized while she is recovering. In the process, she is assaulted and badly bruised. Sophie is left shaken and thereafter never feels safe at home. She barricades herself from the neighborhood. Adding insult to injury, the relatively mild arthritis she has had in her neck for years flares up to cause headaches.

Sophie's children fear for her safety in what is perceived as a deteriorating neighborhood. They worry about her health and feel guilty about their inability to care for her at home. It prompts the consideration of a nursing home. Echoing Dan's story in the last chapter, Sophie reminds her son and daughter that she does not want to be a burden on either of them, or on anyone else for that matter. Fully cognizant of her condition and situation, Sophie herself mentions institutional care and does not object in the least when that option and the sale of her home are seriously discussed. As she explains:

> *Just look at me. Anyone with a brain in her head would think I was crazy to stay in there [her house]. I was very sick and weak and I still can't walk, as you can plainly see. And Rachel [her daughter] . . . well, I couldn't ask her to take care of me. She's busy. She works hard every day in that bakery, God bless her. And my son, how he works! They're beautiful children. So you're sick and they take you to the doctor. You're old and you can't walk . . . so they take you to a place like this. What else can you do? So when Rachel says, "Ma, could we do that?" I says, "Don't worry, you and Jerry [the son] have enough to take care of."*

All the bad fortune alters Sophie's view of life. Her usual cheerful outlook turns to fatalism. According to Sophie, she has always believed that she could control life. She could, if she tried, simply aim for what she wanted, work hard, and get it. But the seemingly inexorable events of the recent past now tell her that destiny cannot be ignored. As Sophie repeats, "If it was meant to be, it was meant to be." Looking back over the years, Sophie now finds that the depression she experienced after breaking her hip and becoming an invalid was the result of a mistaken view of life, the disappointment coming from always expecting the best. She now believes that her original, optimistic view was wrong, covering periods of her life when things only appeared to go her way. She reasons that if she had been a fatalist all along, she would have simply accepted what happened rather than become so upset about it.

> *When it comes to health, what can you do? God willing, you don't get too sick. But, for me, what I didn't know is that something else was in the cards. How can you know? Now I know. But did I know then? If that was meant to be, it was meant to be. The doctors can't do nothing about it either. You can't blame them; you can't blame anyone. You can't blame yourself either. It just wasn't meant to be. That's all. That's what I believe.*

At the same time, Sophie reminds me that, even though she's been placed in a nursing home, she still is grateful. She is thankful for the place where she now lives. She is grateful for the staff, who admittedly give her the best care. She is grateful to the doctors and the therapists who make other "hospitals" where she has been look like poor seconds in comparison. She is grateful for the abundant meals, although, as others do, she complains that sometimes they are not to her liking. While it is not home, it is a good place for an old person who needs constant attention. As she puts it, it is something one "can't really ask a family to do." Her attitude seems altogether realistic and her orientation apparently adjusted to her circumstances. In fact, in the course of making these comments, Sophie points out that she has made a complete adjustment.

Yet, in speaking with Sophie about other aspects of her life, in particular, about family living, filial sentiments, house, and home, her ties, traditions, and troubles take on a different meaning. Sophie has not only experienced chronic illness and presented a burden of care; she also has been a very caring mother and grandmother. In this context, what has happened to her over the last few years amounts to abandonment and the virtual destruction of a house and home. While she does not blame her children for putting her in a place that does have good care, when she thinks about what her family has meant to her and she to them, she becomes very sad, lonely, and disgruntled. It is not only a different context for thinking about what has happened, but also, as she implies, set in a "different mood."

You sometimes get to thinking. You know how you get sometimes. I get that way a lot. You start to think about your family, your children, your home . . . and how you don't see them very much. All you see here are the nurses and the four walls. It's like a prison. You think about your whole life, really. You get into that different mood and things start to look really, really bad and you get really sad.

In this mood, Sophie's assessment of the last few years of her life takes on a decidedly morbid tone, far different from the rational, positive assessment presented regarding her personal adjustment to a fine "hospital." In her morbid mood, ties with her children and grandchildren are depicted as having been torn apart. As she poignantly states, "I feel that my whole life—Rachel, Jerry, and everyone—was just ripped away from me, just like that." She explains that it is the worst thing that could happen in old age, to be taken away from one's family and familiar surroundings. In this mood, the nursing home is not so much a hospital as it is not home. It is a place that represents the exact opposite of what she so achingly longs for. In this mood, Sophie asserts, "This place [the nursing home] can never, never replace what I had before."

These are not just occasions to express longing, but deep feelings. At these times, she weeps painfully. The memory of what Sophie and other patients often call "the little things"—a home's familiar smells, a favorite chair, an annoying neighbor, a flower bed—can charge into the present and transform the most sober demeanor and rational estimate of current circumstances into a gushing forth of distress.

In this mood, Sophie feels profoundly alone, bereft of the only intimate ties she has known. Her conduct and attitude are not ones of positive adjustment and realism, but detachment and isolation. Her children's and grandchildren's dutiful visits seem to make little difference, even while the visits are said to be sobering and assuring at other times. Sophie reports that, in this mood, it is all she can do not to blame her children for what has happened to her. She reports that she feels like a stranger in their presence, even though she cherishes their visits. At worst, she feels abandoned. For all the good the nursing home otherwise seems to do, in this mood it is nothing.

Which is Sophie's story? The version presenting a personal adjustment to institutionalization that occasionally breaks down or the version showing a profound detachment from life? Or is Sophie's a story of fitful shifts in mood? Is Sophie saying that she likes the nursing home but hates it?

Several staff members, notably the social worker and a nurse, as well as a few patients on Sophie's floor believe the latter. To them, Sophie is "moody" or confused, probably an undiagnosed manic depressive. They find her difficult to approach at times, unpleasant to be near because she seems so unpredictable. They cannot understand how someone who has such admittedly wonderful children, who visit her almost daily, can suffer so much from loneliness. At the same time, they cannot see how she can sometimes take what has happened to her in such stride and seem so "totally adjusted," so stoic. The contrast signals a kind of maladjustment in its own right, if not a sickness. To these staff members and others, Sophie has not "really" resolved the challenges of adjusting to institutional living. Indeed, the nurse remarks that Sophie's is a typical case of not being able to face up to reality.

There is another version. Sophie acknowledges the "moods" she alternately takes in thinking about her life before and after institutionalization. Taking serious account of the contexts of her considerations and expressions, it is evident that Sophie's reactions can be seen as the *occasional* pain of longing for home, not symptoms of an underlying maladjustment. In that sense, what Sophie thinks and feels can be conceived as something everyone does and conveys, in their own ways of course, as he or she responds to experience against a background of shifting moods and contrasting visions. In this regard, Sophie's story is less one of a uniformly understood, psychiatric subject than it is about a complex, personal articulation of the opposing themes of hospital and home, finding expressions in different moods. It is a story whose character does not so much exhibit a moral career as a configuration of contrasting, related judgments and sentiments.

Making a New Home: Wilma's Story

In an important article on the psychosocial processes linking person to place, Rubinstein (1989a) argues that individuals utilize publicly shared categories for organizing the meaning of their environments. In reference to the home environment, he writes:

The process of ordering *refers to the way a home environment is structured by an individual according to that person's version of contemporary, external, sociocultural schemata, those that dictate "times and places for entering, entertaining, sleeping, [and] eating" (Werner, Altman & Oxley, 1985) as well as other features of domestic structure (Dovey, 1985). Ordering is an individual's set of ideas about where things go, and it is concerned with tasks such as deciding on room function, furniture placement, and the use of decoration. In this way, sociocultural order is the object of individual interpretation (p. S47).*

In linking public with personal domains of experience, Rubinstein adds to the growing body of literature concerning how individual interpretation is patterned by shared understandings. He simultaneously highlights the distinct environmental marking of individual biography in what is called the "person-centered process."

Rubinstein describes the link between sociocultural order and individual interpretation as rule-like. For example, living rooms are most public and bedrooms most private. As he indicates, "Culture suggests general rules for ordering and arranging space" (p. S47). He does caution that the arrangement of things varies by class and the house form itself. But, while insightful, the conceptualization is still too general and consensual. The way culture is said to affect individual interpretation is all encompassing, as if the rules shared, say, about the privacy of particular spaces, were straightforward and ubiquitous to persons in all circumstances, even while individually adapted and class related. According to Rubinstein, variety comes with the "infinite variations" produced by individuals. There is little sense that certain places, such as hospitals, nursing homes, or prisons, provide their own formal or informal rules concerning the privacy of space, which differ from the rules of other locales. *Local* cultures feature their own public offerings and guidelines for individual application (Gubrium, 1989a; Frost et al., 1985).

What is more, in Rubinstein's formulation, there seems to be no idea that the rules he discusses as available for "infinite" individual adaptation may pose dilemmas for local adherents. In regard to such environmental order as room arrangement, the opposed understandings of the nursing home as a hospital versus a home present conflicting messages about the placement of objects in one's "own" room. Is the message to make the room homey by organizing objects as one desires, or to keep it conducive to high quality professional caregiving? Opposed understandings of time also present conflicting messages about whether one can secure time for privacy separate from the enduring rhythms of organizational time.

The themes of Wilma's story reflect these local cultural contradictions, in particular as they pertain to her attempt to make a new home for herself in Blue Springs, the facility where she is a patient. She is 75 years old, has had several heart attacks, has incapacitating arthritis in her feet, is wheelchair-bound, and has lived at Blue Springs for a year. Her husband was killed in a hunting accident and that, as she remarks, "left me totally and completely alone." She and her husband were only children and had no children of their own. After unsuccessfully trying to make it on her own, she is helped in arranging nursing home placement. Financially secure, she seeks admission to Blue Springs, a facility known to be posh, well managed, and expensive.

At first, Wilma feels she has made a mistake moving there, explaining that it certainly is not anything like home even though "they take pretty good care of you." Wilma is obsessed with thoughts about home, but not the house she shared with her husband for so many years, which she sold quickly enough, placing some of her favorite pieces of furniture in storage "just in case." Rather, her obsession centers on the desire to find a place to live that she can call "home." According to Wilma, in that regard, "Blue Springs doesn't fit the bill." She condescendingly compares the life she believes she can have with the life she now leads. It is not a pretty picture, especially for someone accustomed to "the good things in life." While Wilma is housed in a private room, it "just isn't like home." While she has arranged for a variety of special services such as personal hairdressing and manicuring, it "just isn't" what she is used to. In virtually every respect, it isn't home to her.

Wilma complains, too, about how she feels "cut off" from living at Blue Springs, as if life stood still in the place. She explains that at least when she was in her own home, even after her husband was killed, the things they owned together "kept her going" and made it seem like he was around in some way. Her husband had been an avid hunter. Even after he died, she would look at and touch his hunting gear and clothing, thinking of late autumns and winters when he left for two or three days at a time and returned with ducks or sometimes a deer. The clatter of the neighborhood reminded her of the workaday world. When she heard neighborhood activity in the mornings and afternoons, she knew it was Saturday or Sunday; when she did not, she knew it was a weekday. The absence of these things at Blue Springs now causes her to lose track of time. As other patients and residents mention, "little things," now gone, had their way of keeping memories of a lifetime alive. The afghans she had knit for her own bed and the sofa in the den were always visible in the winter; she put them away during the summer. Little things like the burn marks from her husband's cigarettes on one of her favorite end tables, which she never did get around to repairing, had a way of filling the air with smoke and suggesting that she "get up and make sure he hadn't fallen asleep smoking."

Wilma now finds that all that seems to matter is that time passes and cares are taken care of. One day is like any other. As many patients do, Wilma comments that it really does not matter anyway what day it is or the hour because there is no good reason to keep time. In reference to "her things," she mentions:

> *You know all my stuff is in storage. I did that just in case. When I decide to leave here, at least I'll have my things. All this stuff around here [her room] belongs to the institution. It's their bed, their dresser, their chair, their nightstand. [Points to each in turn.] None of it's mine. But that's okay; it doesn't really matter as long as they [staff] take care of me. If I brought some of my stuff in here . . . like some of the other ladies . . . well, it'd just make me sad because it would remind me too much of him [her husband] maybe. [Long pause.] Methinks I complain too much. [We both laugh.] Maybe it's good because there's nothing in here to remind me of the past . . . or the future! [We both laugh again.]*

Wilma does not actively seek discharge or placement elsewhere. Complaints about the lack of special amenities and the timelessness are balanced with testimonials to the "good care" she receives. Sounding like Sophie, Wilma comments:

> *But it's not all black and white either. It's not home, as I said, but they take care of the patients here. The food . . . well . . . it's awful. But I have to say, too, that you do get three squares a day. As you can see, they provide nice rooms, a nice window, and the furnishings are tasteful. But they just don't compare with my own things. Now there's furniture! [Gives details.] But it's an institution and you really can't expect too much. They're real good about watching over the people. I can't complain about that, really.*

As time passes, Wilma begins to enjoy the company of a *"very nice gentleman down the hall,"* she emphasizes. She has known Jimmy for some time, but did not give him much thought until recently. Jimmy was a resident in a different unit of the nursing home until he fell and broke his hip and later developed a tremor in his hands, which was diagnosed as early Parkinson's. He is moved to one of the patient care units because it is better equipped to meet his needs. Jimmy now takes daily walks with a quad-cane and is mobile enough to make frequent forays outdoors. Wilma remarks that the first clue that he seemed interested in her was when he gave her a small clutch of tulips picked from the side of the building.

This and other signs of affection soon differentially highlight for Wilma the connection between her "little things," home, and time. Recalling Jimmy's initial overture, she comments on how surprised and touched she had been.

> And what do you know? I thought of my lovely vase right away . . . the one with the painted tulips. It was kind of silly, I guess, because I immediately said to Jimmy, "Wait a minute and I'll see if I can find something to put them in." Well, wouldn't you know it, but I started looking for that vase! I was a bit embarrassed, but, of course, I didn't tell him that. [The vase was in storage.] He'd think I was losing my mind. It was just a habit of mine, that I was used to getting it out at home whenever I got flowers. Maybe I was a bit giddy, too, like a schoolgirl? [We both laugh.]

Until her relationship with Jimmy developed, Wilma resigned herself to the rhythms of institutional life, periodically reminiscing about home and longing for her previous life. She literally had put the objects and "little things" of her previous life in storage. However, as her relationship with Jimmy grows, she comes face to face with the nursing home's cultural contradictions.

In the routine details of daily living, Wilma encounters the many ways Blue Springs is not home. As she puts together the semblance of a relationship with Jimmy, with its own developing interpersonal history, she experiences the local routines that serve to treat her and Jimmy as individual patients, not as a couple, and the resistance to allocating them unscheduled time alone. Indeed, Jimmy has been asked sarcastically on a number of occasions why he can no longer be found in his room.

As Wilma looks ahead to Jimmy's attentions and grows fond of his company, her furniture, "little things," and room take on a new significance. They become objects and space she begins to appropriate to a new tie, with Jimmy. When he visits her, she wants to entertain him in *her* room. It is a place for her and him together, not for others. More than ever, she means it to be personal space. As she attempts to secure the privacy of her room, she has to deal with the fact that the space is part of something more nearly hospital-like. It now seems to matter that this is where she, herself, lives. She cherishes Jimmy's visits and entertains him as "royally" as she can, but is annoyed by the institutional intrusions on their time together— the pressure she feels to keep her door open or ajar, the periodic checkups by the nurse's aide, the regular solicitations to bingo and activities, among other reminders of an organizational schedule.

Jimmy eventually proposes marriage and Wilma accepts. Looking forward to Jimmy's moving in with her, Wilma starts to prepare her "home." To the extent permitted, she has a few items of institutional furniture moved out and brings in items she has taken out of storage. She decorates the room with pictures and bric-a-brac, making the room as close to home as possible. She is careful not to move in anything that belonged to her first husband. Jimmy has very little of his own to contribute. He is admittedly not very interested in such things.

Courtship and the project of making a new home are not without their difficulties and resentments. When Jimmy is courting Wilma, several other patients and staff members mock their romance and "what a cute couple" they make. There is frequent and loud speculation about what goes on in the room behind "closed" doors. More than Jimmy, Wilma resents how the couple's intimacies are constant topics of public conjecture and debate. It is bad enough that their personal space often is rudely intruded upon. It is worse to think that she has no privacy at all because her sexuality is a public concern.

Several staff members get into the habit of speaking of the couple as "playing house." The common sentiment is that Jimmy and Wilma are not just a "cute couple," but even as a married couple are still doing things that older people, especially patients, really should not. In staff members' comments, it is evident that even marriage cannot easily contain couplehood and home within the confines of a place where people are not just housed, but are sick, incapacitated, and in need of skilled care.

Against the social consequences of the tensions between home and hospital, Wilma's "housework" is never ending. Just as staff, especially housekeeping and the nurses' aides, move her things around for their convenience and for ostensible purposes of safety, Wilma concertedly moves them back according to her own sense of domestic order. While Jimmy professes disinterest in these matters, Wilma interprets what she takes to be "hints" of his preferences to further prevail on the room's decor. The placement of even the littlest things has personal consequences. As she pointedly comments:

> *Sometimes you get real tired of all the guff you have to take. You can't move somewhere because . . . well, neither of us is able to make it on their own. So you stay put. But it's hard to live together in a place like this. It takes all may energies to just keep my things nice and the place the way we like it. God knows I don't have that much strength. But we'll make it. Whatever it's worth, it's home. As they say, home is where the heart is. [We both laugh.]*

Making Do: Hal's Story

Hal lives in a nursing home, but he is not a patient. He is a resident on John's floor, the man who ran afoul of Phoebe's clique. The consensus among residents is that except for living on the premises of a nursing home, residents are "really" leading a hotel-like existence, taking their meals together in the dining room, but coming and going as they please.

According to Hal, it has never been his desire to take up residence in a "place like this." He explains that, while there is the pretense of residential living, there are many reminders that it is not home. One of the common minor irritations is the medical wrist band each resident is required to wear. There are any number of occasions on which he has been embarrassed as someone on the outside has asked why he is wearing the band. He feels compelled to fib, explaining, for example, that he has just visited a hospital as an outpatient and forgotten to remove it.

Hal is 81 years old, relatively fit, and socially active. His wife, Millie, is gravely ill and a patient on one of the skilled care floors of the nursing home. Hal moved into the facility to be near her. She has had diabetes for years, which has gotten progressively worse in old age. She is now suffering complications, having lost most of her eyesight and developed gangrene in her feet, which have had to be amputated. Millie is in constant pain from festering sores on her legs and, most recently, has been showing signs of confusion.

By and large, the local ties of patients and residents are limited to their immediate floors. There are exceptions, of course. For example, residents who develop medical or psychosocial problems deemed to require nursing care are likely to be transferred to intermediate or skilled care floors, if they wish to remain in the nursing home. Fewer patients, who have recovered sufficiently to no longer warrant nursing care, request transfers to the first floor and become residents. In the process, ties between floors are established, but weaken as localized daily routines and the physical bounds of the environment take effect. Hal is one of the few who has a spouse on another floor. Ties with her and others on another floor combine with his own to form an exceptionally large network of regular acquaintances.

Because Hal's ties cut across levels of care and floors, they present him with unique troubles. Hal encounters the personal dilemmas of the local cultural contradictions of home and hospital as he daily moves about the facility. Hal frequently notes the "difficulty" and "nervousness," as he puts it, he has to face "day in and day out" in keeping track of Millie upstairs, while trying to be cheerful and a regular guy downstairs. Hal's story extends the routine tensions of home versus hospital into the sharp contrasts of wellness and sickness, living and dying, and their related public sentiments. Hal explains:

Did you see Millie this morning? [I reported that I'd seen her and had asked a nurse how she was doing.] That's good. Thanks. You're a good sport. It's not easy . . . going up there day in and day out and seeing her like that. It's pitiful. Poor thing. She's suffering so much and I can't do anything for her . . . Oh, [long pause] I try to keep tabs on how she's treated. I make sure she's taken care of and that the staff is not sitting on their behinds and letting her suffer when she could be getting some relief. But, you know, keeping track of Millie takes its toll, too. You can't imagine how difficult it is and how nervous it makes you. It's

frightening sometimes. It's a real hospital up there and people are sick.
They're suffering and dying. You come down just two floors, on that
elevator there, and it's like moving between two different worlds . . . day
in and day out.

Asked to explain what he means by two different worlds and
his related nervousness, he touches on the personal difficulties of
managing himself in his circumstance:

Naturally, you're nervous because your wife is suffering and you're afraid
for her. You're nervous, too, because down here [on the resident's floor]
you're not supposed to be thinking about sickness and death all the time.
You know, you're a resident. Well, yes, the old ladies do like to talk
about their aches and pains, but that's different. That's gossip and
something to pass the time. It's real for me and it's hard to be cheerful
when, day in and day out, you're faced with all that's happening
upstairs. Put yourself in my place, Jay, and ask yourself how you'd feel.

Hal describes other troubles. At times, the staff on Millie's
floor resent his interference. Hal mentions how careful he has to be
not to complain too much. He fears the aides might retaliate by
taking it out on Millie. He often "bites his tongue," as he grimaces,
when he should actually say something. Hal describes, too, the
trouble his ties to his wife pose for his attempt to "reside" on the
first floor. He cannot simply deal with the daily round of living on
the floor, get involved like the others and leave it at that, because his
wife and life upstairs are constantly on his mind. It is very difficult
to manage, on a daily basis, the sentiments of positive attachment
and involvement alongside the sentiments of impending loss and
social gloom, affective counterparts of home versus hospital.

Hal points out that he has very little control over his mood
and cannot be blamed for how he feels and appears. He describes
how the other residents, while sympathizing with him over his
wife's condition, also consider him to be too morose:

They think I'm gloomy sometimes. You really can't blame them, can
you? It's like this. I go up there and Millie's having a bad day. Well,
right away, I start to feel sad. You know how it is. You feel sad for
them. Their feelings become your feelings. You can't help it. That's
nature, I guess. You know, when you carry someone around in your

heart, you feel it just as if it was you. It's something you can't handle. And, boy, do I know it, too. I just know that if I go up there and find it's one of her bad days, then it's a bad day all around for me.

Hal is not the only resident who contrasts "up there" with "down here," the distinction between life on patient care floors and residential living. It is a commonplace comparison. Still, more than most, Hal lives out the sentimental attachments of the distinction. The distinction goes beyond the territorial; it signals identity. Up there, one is a patient. Up there one resides in a hospital-like setting in the midst of sickness. Down here, one is a resident. To the extent residents are down here, they are simply being at home. Indeed, residents define themselves as much by what they are not as by what they are. They are not patients. In this regard, an enduring trouble for Hal is that these distinctions, which are a ready source of identity for most, constantly challenge each other for him.

Living on a daily basis at the border of home and hospital, Hal experiences a brand of the local temporal tension felt by Sophie, Wilma, and others. While there are patients like Wilma, who attempt to establish new pasts and futures, and like Sophie, who occasionally long for an old past, Hal's reflection on life up there presents it as timeless. He remarks that up there, time seems to stand still. There is no past because all that matters is one's current pain and suffering. Neither is there a future up there, which makes Hal nervous and fearful when thinking about Millie.

Asked how he handles all these contrasts, Hal responds, "You make do." In explaining what he means, it is evident that making do entails working at experiential containment. Even though he is very sad while he is up there, he tries his best to keep his feelings under control so that they do not get the best of him when he departs. When Hal leaves the nursing home on various errands, he simply attempts to be the resident he is. In fact, each time, he tries his best to bring Millie a little news of home and the neighborhood, "to get her mind off all the sickness." He takes the bus to visit lifelong friends rather than encouraging them to visit him at the nursing home. He feels they would probably not want to set foot in such a place if it were not necessary. He understands perfectly how they feel; he feels the same way about having to visit upstairs in the nursing home.

Millie does not always recognize Hal when he visits. But Hal talks to her of home and outside matters anyway. As he explains, "She's a human being, too, no matter what she seems to be there in bed and she needs to know that we all care about her." It is his way of bringing home to her, of reminding her that, even while she is gravely ill, she is still part of his own and others' lives, not just the occupant of a sickroom.

Hal's enduring ties with Millie's floor gives him a special function downstairs. He brings news of former residents who have been transferred upstairs. Since many residents avoid going up there because it depresses them, they depend on Hal and a few others to keep abreast of acquaintances' daily lives on other floors. Of course, along with this comes news of illness, suffering, hospitalization, and death. While these conditions occur to some degree on the residential floor, there they signal the troubles of old age as much as they represent institutionalization. In the context of "up there," they are daily reminders of what residents can become—patients—which forecast troubles of their own.

Being Demented: Paul's Story

Paul is one of the growing number of patients in nursing homes with Alzheimer's disease. Until the early eighties, when Alzheimer's became the so-called disease of the century, patients showing symptoms of senile dementia commonly were diagnosed CVA (cerebral vascular accident or stroke) and OBS (organic brain syndrome) if they had no coexisting physical debilities. There probably always were Alzheimer's disease patients in nursing homes. It only has been in the last 10 years that their diagnosis has been the subject of widespread concern regarding special services and unit allocation. In that regard, Paul's story is not particularly new.

Paul's room is located on a skilled care unit of a nursing home. There are patients with a variety of other diagnoses in the immediate vicinity of his room. Like Millie, some have severe complications of diabetes. Like Wilma, some have suffered heart attacks. Some have had strokes and are partially paralyzed. Some have slurred or incomprehensible speech. A few, like Wilma's new husband Jimmy, have symptoms of Parkinson's. Others are bedridden

and rarely, if ever, are seen outside their rooms. Many are physically disabled. A significant number are lucid.

Paul occupies a room immediately adjacent to the nurses' station because floor staff likes to "keep an eye on him." Paul is a "wanderer," meaning that he loses track of his whereabouts. He occasionally walks into others' rooms and, according to a few of the women on the floor, "scares us half to death." Rarely, he "escapes," which means that he somehow finds his way into another unit. He has never wandered outdoors, although there are patients like Paul who have.

Paul's wandering and "restlessness" occasionally cause the staff to restrain him. At times, he can be found secured in a geriatric chair, which is like a highchair for adults. At other times, he is fastened to his bed, writhing to free himself of arm and leg restraints. Paul tends to be very loud when he is restrained. As some patients mention, the restraints "set him off." They aren't sure if it is better to tolerate a restrained Paul yelling at the top of his lungs or a quiet Paul who, at any time, might wander into their rooms. Neither is the staff.

There is a variety of opinion about Paul's intrusions into others' lives on the floor. Some patients cannot understand why the nursing home admits what are believed to be mental patients. To them, Paul is at the peak of physical health—wiry, strong, energetic, ambulatory, "ruggedly good looking," and dexterous. As an LPN on the floor once remarked, "To look at him, you'd think absolutely nothing was wrong with him." To many, this suggests only one thing: Paul has "completely lost his marbles." As Phoebe describes John, Paul is *non compos mentis*.

At the same time, Paul is occasionally the source of much hilarity. His rugged good looks are the butt of jokes and gossip among some patients about how certain women on the floor "really" want Paul to sneak into their rooms "for a good see." Paul's "antics" cause an equal amount of gossip and joking among staff. To staff, he basically is harmless, not at all violent, and in his own confused way, a "gentle giant." In this regard, what staff see in Paul is a man who, when he is not being too difficult, brings variety to their lives.

Paul displays a kind of incoherent conviviality. He regularly ambles over to the nurses' station and wants to "talk over" things. When staff take the time, particularly in the relative quiet of the afternoon, they mimic gossiping with him about whatever they believe to be on his mind. While they cannot understand him, it is evident to them that he thoroughly enjoys their company. When he laughs, they laugh with him.

One of the favored places for observing the goings-on of daily life in a nursing home is the nursing station. Staff and patients often gather around one or patients are collected into the area in their wheelchairs. When Paul is not sleeping, restrained, or otherwise indisposed, he usually can be found near the station on his unit.

In doing fieldwork on Paul's unit, I fondly recall the many times Paul would casually place his elbow on top of the station, chest-level for him and, in his affable way, ask glowingly, "How's life, partner?" From previous experience, I knew that whatever I said in response would not be followed by anything immediately comprehensible. Nevertheless, partly through courtesy and partly because his greeting was so charming, I regularly responded in kind. "Fine partner. How's life been treating you?" I once poured him a plastic cup of water in the process, because he seemed a bit parched. I had been drinking the same while taking field notes. He took the cup, half toasted me, and slugged it back, as if it were a stiff drink. He immediately smiled, gently slammed the cup on the top of the station, and stated with evident pleasure, "That hit the spot." I poured him another. After that, we made a habit of it, combining what seemed to be the semblance of conviviality with the non sequiturs of his dementia. For me, it was a tender and welcome moment each time it occurred. For staff, it was a source of good-humored teasing about how Paul and Jay went drinking in the afternoon.

Given Paul's dementia, is it possible to speak of his ties, traditions, and their related troubles? Certainly, his erratic "ties" in the nursing home cause some difficulty. But are the ties in any way meaningful to Paul, such that it might reasonably be concluded that his version of ties, traditions, and troubles present a story?

Paul's wife, Adele, often "speaks" with, and for, Paul. Her frequent visits with Paul at the nursing home, like my own participation in his self-presentation and self-management in the drink-sharing, does articulate a kind of story. Adele not only speaks her own mind to Paul, but audibly conveys for him what she believes to be his thoughts and feelings. When she finds him restrained, she sometimes approaches the nurses' station and, sympathizing with the staff about the occasional need for this in Paul's case, asks whether they know how he must be feeling, tied to his chair or bed. As she once explains:

> *I know the poor fellow doesn't like it. You can just hear him. He feels like you've put him in jail. He doesn't understand how this could happen to him. When I'm in there, I know that deep down inside, he's asking how anyone could do this to him. Can't we maybe let him stand up and stretch a bit? I know he was pretty bad this morning. I'll watch him.*

I have overheard and actually found myself participating in a number of "conversations" that Adele has with her husband. Joining in, I find myself embellishing the flow of personal and interpersonal logic that she, by speaking for him, articulates as his. In turn, she speaks her own piece. One time, for example, as Adele's conversation with (for) Paul indicates that he is distressed about his relations with others in the nursing home, I find it reasonable to ask him what the source of his troubles is. Without using the exact term, I ask him whether his "ties" with certain persons are causing him to be annoyed and agitated. Adele responds for him, in a manner that seems to follow. I then answer in a compatible fashion. The "conversations" are not always consensual. There are "disagreements," such as when Adele infers that I am misinterpreting what Paul is thinking. The disagreements, nonetheless, lead to corrections that are comprehensible in the flow of exchanges. The organization of conversation itself gives a lucid tenor to all contributions (Sudnow, 1972).

Paul's version of a developing story is not just a discursive ritual performed by Adele, Paul, myself, and others. It can have a moral imperative. The staff know that when Paul allegedly feels wronged, Adele complains bitterly about it. They know Paul is sorrowful because Adele informs them of it. They know when he is being left alone too much and that he, like any human being, needs the company and affection of others, because Adele tells them for him. With others' discursive support and conversational indulgence, Adele keeps Paul's mind and spirit socially alive and working, preserving both by speaking and acting for him (Gubrium, 1986b).

Paul's assigned thoughts and feelings reflect the local cultural contradictions of the nursing home. Adele expresses distress for him when she "knows" Paul feels frightened in the company of strangers. She wants him to feel that this is home, or at least as much like home as possible under the circumstances. She repeatedly reminds others, both staff and patients, that Paul has a past. Thus, she stands as his sentry against the intrusions of the organizational present. She speaks of what he was, has accomplished in life, and how much others have admired him for it. She recounts his foibles and transgressions, too, and uses the information to account for his present conduct. In practice, Paul has a living past. Adele makes sure of that. She publicly maintains his biography, using it to dilute the thrust of the present, its formal roles, and its consequences.

One time, Paul is particularly restless and causes what the nurses' aides describe as a lot of trouble on the AM shift. After being dressed, he wanders about, arbitrarily entering other patients' rooms. Later that day, he insists on having long, drawn-out conversations with several of the men on the floor. They complain that Paul does not make any sense and irritates them. This is reported to Adele. She sympathizes as always. When the nurse warns her that he will have to be restrained if he continues to bother others and is discourteous, Adele remarks that the nurse is wrong to think that. Adele explains that Paul has "always, always" been a gentleman and "wouldn't dream" of being discourteous to anyone, that it is not "his way" to be like that. She goes on to describe the old Paul in considerable detail, publicly reclaiming Paul's past. Adele cautions the nurse not to blame Paul for what happened because Adele knows that deep down inside Paul would be very upset if he realized what the others thought he was doing. Adele adds, "That's why he gets so upset when you restrain him; he can't imagine that he deserves that."

While in theory Paul is an individual, as a person he cannot be separated from those around him. This, of course, is true for all people—frail elderly, families, and others. What makes Paul's story particularly significant in this regard is that it vividly shows that ties, traditions, and troubles, like other categories of real life, do not belong to individuals, but are assigned to them. People act and respond in terms of what is conveyed to them and what they receive from others in stories. To the extent stories are kept alive, the practical meaning in life is preserved for better or worse, however senseless it might appear to be in theory. As stories are enlivened for others, so is the meaning of their troubles, ties, and traditions. Even the related activity, thoughts, and intentions of the demented are meaningful in stories.

Implications for the Professional Caregiver

The opposed understandings of home versus hospital and the competing temporal logics of organizational time and life history are constant features of the affairs of those who participate in institutional life. One does not simply deal with their pressures and organizational conditions and move on with life. Neither does one simply succumb to, or embrace, one or the other pole of the cultural opposites to become either a complete individual or a complete patient. Even Paul, who is demented, is not just a patient but is preserved biographically by his wife Adele. Her actions mediate home and hospital and organizational time and life history.

While select individual stories do show evidence of differential adherence to one pole or the other, there are constant local imperatives for movement in the opposite direction. Individual memories and the ideology of home living sustain the imperative of one pole, just as organizational rhythms and job restrictions impel one to the opposite pole. Local cultural conditions and individual interests sustain the tension.

CULTURALLY-SENSITIVE INTERVENTION

An implication for the professional caregiver is that one cannot simply attempt to deal with patients or residents in terms of individual adjustment. The idea of adjustment implies that those under consideration become more or less attuned to organizational definitions and rhythms as individuals. Rather than offering counseling in the traditional sense of advice on how to deal with and resolve troubles, professionals should encourage efforts to establish a personally satisfactory balance between the organizational imperatives facing patients and residents. Professionals need to provide culturally sensitive intervention, not to confront institutional life but to validate the inventive ways in which themes of home and life history are articulated and differentially managed.

DEINDIVIDUALIZING ADJUSTMENT

The professional worker who attempts to understand patient lives in terms of personal adjustment places the responsibility for well-being squarely on the patient's shoulders. If one is not adjusting, something is wrong with the patient, especially when he or she has had all the support needed to make an adjustment. Serious consideration of local cultural contradictions suggests that, within certain limits, patients and residents face opposing definitions of personhood and daily living that are broader than the individual. In this regard, the "individual" problems the professional caregiver encounters are cultural. An awareness of this challenges the professional worker to consider the social complexity of a real world that both produces and contains troubled and troublesome lives, separate from individual shortcomings and disabilities, and to deindividualize the concept of adjustment (Mills, 1963).

CHAPTER 6

The Family and the Nursing Home

To adapt a phrase used by Fischer and others (1990), "concern without commitment" may be sign of delimited interest in families' relations with institutionalized elderly. In some eyes, visits are not necessarily indicative of a caring attitude. This contrasts with a common belief that the well-being of the institutionalized exists in direct proportion to the frequency of visitation or the size of the patient's social network, among other quantifications.

The stories in this chapter show that the goings-on of visits are related to diverse ties and traditions, such as a history of volatile interpersonal relations. What has been played out in domestic life outside the nursing home is repeated in, or lurks in the background of, visitation. In the real world, neither visitation nor extended family relations with the nursing home and patient exists in a social or historical vacuum. The quality of relations between the institutionalized and their families is anything but uniformly linear.

Families as Interlopers

There is an important sense in which family members are interlopers in the daily affairs of the nursing home. Families intrude into activities that otherwise have a social logic of their own. This is not to say that they have no official business there, only that it is often felt by family members themselves, staff, patients, and residents that "things are different" with families about. Nursing homes may have visiting hours, time set aside for family members and others to freely enter to see residents. Having hours informs all that there are occasions when outsiders belong on the premises and occasions when they do not. Even without specified visiting hours, the daily organizational rhythms of nursing homes, especially activities associated with different workshifts, have an informal way of making facilities more inviting to outsiders at certain times than others.

Family members are to some extent like strangers on the premises, even while some have a habit of being there daily for extended periods of time. Strangers take stock of things in a way natives do not. Strangers do not take as much for granted (Simmel, 1950: 402–408). They inspect environs for what seems or does not seem right or routine, according to the sense of order they bring with them. Yet the stranger is circumspect, too, in that he or she is aware of his or her own presence, which presents the question of how much the stranger's concern itself is the source of what is observed or encountered.

The family member is also a potential agent for the patient or resident. While some families may be considered lax in this regard, in principle they are initially taken to have a special tie to the patient, signifying loyalty and protection. When the circumspection and concern of the stranger combine with advocacy, the interloper becomes a sentry of care, a potentially formidable intruder.

An enduring theme in this regard relates to the question of how to respond to what is seen or heard as a visiting family member. Should one complain? Will a complaint be taken seriously? Will it show a lack of understanding of institutional routine? Dare one chance repercussions to the resident, or becoming a complainer and eventually being ignored?

The stories of this chapter feature the everyday organizational dilemmas of the interloper. The dilemmas work in tandem with diverse interpersonal traditions to present a mosaic of concern.

Possessive Vigilance: Eula's Story

In some eyes, Eula's care for her husband Henry is a study in total devotion. Henry had a series of strokes that left him disabled and with impaired speech. Eula dutifully cared for him at home for close to 10 years. He became more and more confused, and lost control over bodily functions. While Eula found it difficult to care for him, she admittedly reaped considerable pleasure from being useful. Even before Henry became grossly disabled, she had suspected that because of her small stature and his large physique, she might one day not be able to manage him on her own. It had worried her over the years. But as long as Henry was aware that he needed to help, she remained stoic.

That did not last forever. When he became confused, forgetful, and helpless, she panicked. Eventually, she sought nursing home care. As Eula explains:

> When Henry couldn't help me move him to the wheelchair any more and he wasn't able to help me get him into bed, I was at a total loss. Just look at me. I'm a small woman. Henry's a very heavy man. I would panic. [Details her reactions.] How was I going to move him? I even dropped him once when I tried to lift him out of bed and I just started to cry. It really scared me. I wanted to call for help but I had to hold onto him or he'd slip and break his neck or something. That's when I began to think that I just wasn't strong enough to care for him alone. As long as he was able to help me, I could take care of everything . . . and I did. But when he went limp on me, what else could I do?

Eula's concern followed Henry into the nursing home. She now dutifully and caringly cleans him whenever he "messes up," Eula repeats. Finding that Henry has urinated or defecated in his pants, she tends to him immediately. While she cannot be at his side during breakfast and lunch, she brings him fresh fruit later in the day and soothingly presses each piece to his lips as she whispers tenderly for him to open his mouth and chew carefully. She bakes bread and offers him his favorite end pieces from each loaf, although she knows that she has to be extra cautious in feeding it to him because he easily chokes on dry food. With the help of the aides, she dresses him warmly to go outdoors, places him in a wheelchair, and takes him for walks in the vicinity. She never goes far because she is afraid that if he slips in the chair, she will not be able to reposition him on her own.

Henry's bodily care always has preoccupied Eula. Just as Eula had difficulty turning, lifting, and transferring Henry at home, she now does not believe that "the girls," as she calls the nurses' aides, can manage much better, even though she agrees that as a team they make do. Still, Eula admittedly worries about Henry as never before. Her concern is complicated by a tradition of protective, if not possessive, affection. Eula remarks as she combs Henry's hair:

> Believe you me, Henry and I have never had trouble being close to one another. We was always just so lovey-dovey. He was always stroking my hair and rubbing my back. Pardon me for sayin' this, but I just couldn't ever keep my hands off him. It was like . . . well, like we was always just curled up around each other. Even after he had his strokes and couldn't move around much, I hugged and kissed him all the time. I got a kick out of dressing him and helping him to the bathroom. I felt real close when I could do all those things for him . . . real close. He was my Henry. [She looks at Henry affectionately.] He's still my big baby. Aren't you honey? She kisses and hugs him. [He doesn't respond.]

Finished with what she terms "fussing over him," she talks about the relationship between the affection and Henry's physical management. She repeats that she gets a "kick" out of caring for Henry. She makes it clear that affection is a central theme of their lives, as she puts it, "one of the biggest things for both of us." She is quick to point out that, just because Henry now lives at Green Manor, things have not changed. She still has a need to be close to him, even though she knows that the "girls" can handle his medications and most of his daily physical needs.

There is something exclusive about Eula's concern for Henry's physical management. For Eula, handling him bodily is the sign of a very special relationship, one shared exclusively with Henry over the many years of their marriage. She does not mind others feeding him, even though she knows that the treats she provides him daily are more nutritious than what the nursing home offers. She does mind others dressing and handling him. Dressing him, to her, is different from cleaning him after he has soiled himself. In her mind, cleaning has more to do with sanitation than physical appearance and bodily well-being.

Eula finds it difficult to explain her concern about others' physical contact with her husband. It is not touch so much or the particular body part that she is sensitive about, but what Eula perceives as the function of the physical contact. Any contact required to maintain cleanliness is acceptable. Any contact showing the slightest evidence of physical attraction is taboo. That kind of contact is exclusively Eula's territory.

Eula remarks that her feelings about this have been the source of some tension with others for years and now causes trouble with the aides.

Them girls [aides] is okay. They have it rough and they get pushed around a lot and don't get paid much for it either. They take care of Henry pretty good. But like I said, I don't like them fussin' with him too much. Some things is none of their goddamn business. [I mention the variety of cares completed when she is not around.] Yeah, I know. Well I can't be here all the time. They don't like us to come in very early. But I get him ready for bed. I get him real dolled up in his pajamas and fuss over his hair and stuff. I just love doin' for him like that there. We was always real close. [Whispers.] We used to dress each other up sometimes. I got a real kick out of it. Henry used to say that my body belonged to him and I used to tell him that I owned his body and would do whatever I liked with it. [We both laugh.] I told them girls that a couple of times and they didn't like it. Well, they can shove it.

According to the aides, Eula is very touchy when it comes to handling Henry. They feel Eula appreciates what they do for him, but suspect she thinks she can do better. That does not bother them as much as her constant meddling in physically handling him. As one of the aides comments:

If you ask me, she's too touchy. Sometimes, she comes here and she just drives you crazy . . . like she wants to take over. You start to, like, transfer him [Henry] and just like that [whips her arm] she's up and trying to do it with you. She can really be a pest. It gets to be, like, you really don't want her around when you have to work on him. You know what she said to me? Get this. Like I was giving Henry a back rub and she says to me that that's none of my business and that she'd do it. That woman told me that he gets all the affection he needs from her. Christ! I wasn't giving affection! Is she batty?

Eula's concern sometimes spills over into a vigilance for the bodily cares of other men. She is not as interested in the female residents. According to Eula, what "naturally" can happen between a man and a woman cannot as easily occur between women. The aides resent this. Several complain that how they organize and manage the care of residents is not any of Eula's business. They become particularly upset when they learn that Eula has suggested to other families and the administration that the aides are not handling residents with the proper respect. One aide complains, "It's bad enough when you get shit from some of them, but when you get shit from Haley [a charge nurse] about it too, it hurts."

Eula's story as an interloper in the affairs of Green Manor Nursing Home is not just about vigilance and protectiveness. In some versions, she is a kindly and concerned wife. Staff admire her loyalty and dutiful attention. Some speculate about how care in general might be improved if other families showed equal concern. Eula's visitations are exemplary in that regard. But in the domain of bodily cares, where Eula is ever vigilant, her visits can be admittedly "a pain in the neck." When the balance of her interpersonal relations with the staff tilts in that direction, she is said to be "just awful."

Trying To Be There: Maxine's Story

Maxine's father, Luke, is a patient in the same nursing home. According to a number of aides, she hardly ever visits him. In contrast to staff's periodic complaints about Eula's vigilant, yet concerned presence, Maxine's overall attitude is said to be glib and uncaring.

Maxine infers as much from a variety of related comments. When she urges the activity director to get her father involved in recreation and the passive range of motion exercises available three afternoons a week, the director comments on the difficulty of "getting them [patients] going" without the cooperation and support of the family. As Maxine is Luke's only family, she takes this to be a statement about her lack of concern. When Maxine asks the charge nurse on the floor, in what Maxine believes is a civil manner, how well her father is eating and whether he continues to be constipated, the nurse's response is curt. Maxine interprets this to be the result of the nurse reading Maxine as believing that Luke is not well cared for. Sensitive to this, Maxine responds, to no avail, that the question is simply meant to inquire about her father's health.

Luke has been a patient at Green Manor for 14 months. In that time, he has become the unit staff's pet. They readily respond to his kindly manner. While he suffers from emphysema and remains in his bed or in the immediate vicinity of his room most of the time, Luke nonetheless is habitually cheerful and funny. The aides see to it that he is up in his wheelchair when he is willing and able. His cheerfulness is contagious. A number of staff members on the floor note that if they feel a bit "down," all they have to do is walk into Luke's room and he has kind and understanding words for them. As one of the aides reports:

> *He's a very, very nice man. God! Give me Luke any day instead of my old man! He's like a father to the girls. I've been working here for about five months and I can tell you it's people like him that make you think twice before quitting. [I asked her to explain.] Oh, it's the way he puts things. He really never complains like some of the other patients, but you know when he doesn't think you're doing the right thing. It's like you know he thinks a lot of the girls and knows the pressures we're all under and all the crud you have to take in a place like this. When you have all this gloom and sickness around you all the time, you can get pretty down. It's just nice to have someone like him around.*

Others mention that it is the way Luke "comes across"; his attitude makes the difference. He is not gushy like some of the women on the floor, who are said to be nice only when a favor is needed. He does not patronize the aides just because they do not have the education or background he does. And he is not rude to the black and Asian aides. He treats them all alike.

It is generally believed that people go out of their way to do things for Luke. Aides peek into his room on the way down the hall and greet him in good humor, whether or not he is formally part of their caseload. Almost every afternoon, relatives of patients who have come to know and admire Luke make a point of talking with him. The activity director says that she "loves to have him around," but knows, too, that she has to take care not to encourage him too much because of his difficulty breathing. Maxine feels at times that the staff thinks they actually own Luke.

While Maxine welcomes the staff's attention to, and their admiration for, her father, she worries about things, especially whether her sometimes overbearing attitude is backfiring. She complains that the staff make her think they will "bite off her head" if she dares mention anything related to the quality of his care. She feels caught between wanting to know how her father is doing and remaining silent so as not to offend staff members' sensibilities. Maxine knows the nursing staff is not fond of her; at the same time, she needs to make sure Luke gets all the attention he requires.

Of equal concern to Maxine are competing demands on her time that keep her away from her father. She owns and operates a fashionable women's clothing store in town, spending long hours there. The business exhausts her. While she has been divorced for many years, has no children and thus few domestic obligations, at the end of the day she feels she needs to "just get home, kick off my shoes, and collapse." This competes with her desire to see her father.

Maxine loves Luke. Until he was physically incapacitated, she drew constant inspiration from the example he set at work. Luke was a full, working partner in the business. She misses his companionship, loyalty, and leadership. Whenever she visits him at the nursing home, she not only extends the quiet affection that always characterized their relationship but relishes his continuing good counsel and total devotion to her.

The nursing staff are aware of the family business. Many have passed by the store at one time or another. Few have sufficient income to purchase anything. Some of the aides resent Maxine for her association with what they cannot have. As one once blurts:

> She's really something, that gal. She comes in here and sniffs around like she owns the place. It just makes you sick sometimes . . . all that expensive stuff she's got on. You can just see big bucks all over her. It's her Miss High Fashion attitude that makes you just mad as hell. She comes in here real quick-like and wants to know what's going on . . . like we're not doing our job or something. And what's she do? She's just being fancy all day. Well, I'm not going to work my buns off for her and have her come in here and act like I'm a rug to walk on. No sir.

As far as the aides are concerned, Maxine has it "too good" and has nothing to complain about. The mere suggestion that Maxine really works is taken to be nonsense, if not outright pretension. Maxine's concern for Luke is perceived likewise.

Aware of staff's feelings about her, Maxine nonetheless believes that, in her own way and under the circumstances, she is doing the best she can for her father. She touchingly cries that she wishes she could do more. In talking about her competing obligations, her father's care, and staff resentment, Maxine reports that she always tries to be there for Luke, at his side whenever he needs her.

Maxine feels caught in a dreadful dilemma. On one side, the intimate tie she has with her father, secured in lifelong companionship, sustains a genuine concern for his welfare despite staff's perception of a contrary attitude. Yet, to the staff, the nature of her visits shows that Maxine could care less. On the other side, her attempt to optimize the time she spends with her father, not only visiting but, at the same time, expeditiously inquiring about his care, makes her seem gruff, glib, and specious. Because Maxine is viewed as wanting everything done at once and "her way," she is thought to be interested only in the mechanics of her father's care, not its spirit.

Maxine is a different kind of interloper than Eula. The trouble Eula causes the nursing staff centers on the care surrounding her husband's physical management; the troubles Eula reaps in return are linked with the kind of relationship she has formed with her husband over the years. Otherwise Eula is perceived as a dutiful and indulgent wife. In contrast, even while Maxine and Luke have an intimate interpersonal history, Maxine is considered to be totally self-centered and perfunctory, her behavior during visits being a clear sign of her character. While Eula causes trouble for staff at times, Maxine is considered to be, simply, "a bitch." As one of the aides once bitterly remarks after Maxine leaves for the evening:

> Why does she pretend that she's interested? She's only interested in herself and she hassles everyone around her just to make herself look good . . . like she wants to show us she cares about the old man. You wonder sometimes how such a sweetie [Luke] could have such a bitch for a daughter. Just look at how she acts when she's around—a bitch. Miss High and Mighty. You just know she thinks she's too good for us. I can see right through her and I don't think she's really that interested in him [Luke] either.

However the sentiments of the various parties to Luke's care are judged, it is evident that the sentiments are entangled with broader ties and traditions. Maxine, for one, realizes that no matter how dutiful her visits to her father, she is never simply a daughter, more or less present in the nursing home. Her presence is mediated by the ascribed meaning of her absence and her presumed attitude.

Going Through the Motions?: Herb's Story

Following her husband's death, Thelma's home falls into considerable disrepair. Her son, Herb, thinks it best to sell the house, persuading his mother she would better off living upstairs from him. Herb's wife, Elaine, finds no compelling reason not to agree to the arrangement. The upstairs apartment is separate enough to keep everybody happy, yet close enough to check on Thelma conveniently.

It is an ideal arrangement until Thelma begins to lose her memory. The woman that Herb describes as a formerly sober and independent person forgets to do the "littlest things," like closing the windows during rainstorms and turning off the gas stove. A number of times, water drips downstairs from an overflowing bath-tub because of what Herb calls his mother's negligence. Herb discovers his mother wandering outdoors during the night, ostensibly because the dog has been left in the yard and wants to be let in. Herb and Elaine do have a pet poodle, but Herb is always careful, he claims, to see that the dog is indoors at night. By his own reckoning, Herb is a fastidious and conscientious person with a keen sense of responsibility and much pride of ownership. He would never make such a mistake, let alone ignore the weather and the damage it can do to a house.

Thelma is diagnosed with Alzheimer's. Herb learns all he can about the disease. As Elaine reports, "He's the kind of person who likes everything in its place and now he's making a full-time job of looking into Alzheimer's." Elaine "just knows" that if Herb had been a doctor, he would have had the disease cured by now. The zeal Herb showed at work before he retired and in his domestic affairs throughout his life simply is transferred to dealing with his mother's difficulties. Whatever project Herb takes on, he dispatches efficiently.

Herb joins a local support group for family caregivers. He meets caregivers whose families are deeply troubled by the disease's interpersonal effects. It has caused strains in many marriages and "bad feelings" between family members. Other caregivers have not been affected this way. Neither has Herb. His relations with Elaine remain cordial and secure. Rarely, if ever, are they infringed upon by Thelma's behavior. Rather, what drives Herb's attention to the effects of the disease is the havoc his mother's behavior increasingly wreaks on the temporal and physical order of his household.

As support group proceedings do, participants share their thoughts and feelings about home care. Herb likewise contributes, dwelling on the practical consequences of changes in his mother's conditions. Some participants, however, are annoyed that, for Herb, there is no indication that he is "going through it" as a person, as it is said one normally does in such matters. The facilitator remarks:

> *You know, Herb, sometimes I get the impression that, to you, it's [his mother's behavior] all a matter of what she's doing to your house. Aren't you feeling something? Aren't you going through something? I know you're concerned with what's happening to Thelma, but you might ask yourself if it's really her you're concerned about or that she's messing up the house all the time. We all know that you take care of things better than anyone and see to your mother's comfort and safety better than any parent deserves. But deep, down inside, you know you're feeling something, aren't you? We all go through it.*

In the early stages of home care, caregivers are said to dwell on cure and the well-being of the patient, ignoring their own needs. Only much later in the process of adjustment is there a stage of self-concern experienced by the caregiver. The stages pertain to the caregiver's feelings as much as to caregiving priorities. The problem is that Herb is perceived as having no feelings about the matter, nor are his priorities viewed to be correct.

Herb does not take offense at the response. He accepts comments as a regular part of the group's proceedings, responding to questions about where he "is at" (referring to the place of his feelings in the overall process of personal adjustment) with answers rooted in a continuing concern with domestic order.

This does not much change as Herb, some time later, considers placing Thelma in a nursing home. Even in the alleged later stages of adjustment to home care, Herb is exceptional. Bothering the other participants of the support group, in particular the facilitator, is the fact that there is not even a sign of an adjustment problem "at the end," meaning just before institutionalizing his mother. Is Herb so callous as just to be going through the motions of caring?

As Herb conveys it, an initial interest in learning how to manage the Alzheimer's disease victim at home gradually has shifted to a careful consideration of care options when caregiving at home is no longer feasible. For Herb, it is now time to restore order to the household. In a particularly telling comment, he remarks that "it never, ever really had that much to do" with how he felt, but

> *for me, she . . . yeah she's my mother, but when a person can't live with you like a person and come and go like a human being, then something has to be done. I could see it from the very beginning. At first, she just messed up a bit. Well, you don't gripe about things like that. You just take care of it. But when I started to think that she was really losing her mind, she really has to be in a place that can handle all the stuff she does. It never, ever really had that much to do with how I felt about her. I always loved my mother and I still love her. I just can't see that anyone can live like that.*

Herb eventually places his mother in what is claimed to be the finest nursing home in the area. He drops out of the Alzheimer's disease support group and joins the nursing home's support group for families. The latter is the pride of the facility's social worker. In biweekly meetings, participants are introduced to a range of family issues: what to look for in continuing care, how to listen to the patient ("active listening"), and how to make the best of nursing home visits ("effective visitation"), among other matters.

Herb again encounters the theme of personal adjustment. Of primary interest in the nursing home support group is postplacement adjustment. It is assumed that placement does not end the family's reaction to events surrounding institutionalization. Following placement, family members' feelings are said to change in a recognizable fashion, again occurring in stages.

Like the facilitator of the first support group, the nursing home's social worker figures Herb's "adjustment" to be problematic. Herb is not going through the various stages, only "going through the motions," the same expression the facilitator had used. Separately, the social worker explains to me that Herb does not have any feelings about the situation. All that seems to interest him is that the details of his life are in order. Diagnostically, the social worker states that Herb is keeping his feelings in and missing the opportunity to vent and resolve his distress. She warns that hidden, festering emotions have a way of bursting forth, when it may be too late to do anything about them.

Herb never does offer explicit psychosocial adjustment material, although there are numerous readings of what he allegedly is going through "underneath it all." The social worker is frustrated because she cannot readily use the categories and techniques she has learned or developed to deal with his adjustment. At the same time, Herb often mentions how much he loves his mother, which indicates to the social worker that there "must" be deep and old emotional ties between them. The social worker does not believe he is lying or just "putting on the dog," as she remarks. She adds, "Why should he keep coming to see her [the mother] when she doesn't even recognize him anymore and why should he even come to the meetings?" Herb's regular visits to the home, his dutiful participation in the family program, and the questions he routinely asks about his mother, suggest to the social worker that he cares. She sums it up by saying that Herb's is a "valiant," but unfortunate attempt to go through the motions, made possible by the fact that he is very good at covering his feelings.

Lengthy discussions with Herb reveal that he has a different interpretation, one he has maintained all along. While the local cultures of both support groups he has attended take affective ties and changing feelings to be an inextricable feature of interpersonal relations, especially in matters of filial responsibility, Herb separates feelings from responsibility. It always has been his belief that one does not tinker with love, affection, and feelings by "talking them to death," as he puts it. Love and affection are things that just happen or are lost in the course of people's dealings with one another. Herb gives priority to things about which something can be done. He participated in the home care support group because he needed to know how to keep his mother comfortable and safe. It was his lessening ability to assure this on his own that prompted him to place her in a nursing home. He now participates in the nursing home support group because it keeps him apprised of how his mother is faring in comparison to other patients. Herb explains that none of this is a matter of changing feelings about her.

Conjuring Up Old Hostilities: Pearl's Story

Pearl's mother, Marie, is a patient in the same nursing home as Thelma, Herb's mother. The two mothers do not know each other. Their rooms are in separate units and, except for infrequent excursions beyond their immediate environs, each remains in the vicinity of her room. Pearl visits her mother in the evening, once or twice a week.

According to staff, the visits are decidedly emotional and have a pattern. Each begins relatively cheerfully. Pearl greets the staff in the lobby and chats a bit about the day's happenings. Major events are recounted—recent deaths, employee turnover, humorous and unfortunate occurrences. Pearl is particularly fond of the affable receptionist, who rarely misses the opportunity to fill Pearl in on the latest local news. Pearl carries the good humor to her mother's room, warmly greeting those whom she meets along the way.

When I first meet Pearl and observe her interactions with Marie, I marvel at how patient Pearl can be with her mother. Pearl maintains her composure and pleasantly forges on even when Marie is irritable. When Marie is withdrawn and refuses to speak, Pearl persists in drawing out her mother.

When I first mention to several staff members and a few patients that Pearl's good cheer and apparent indulgence of her mother are remarkable, I am told that I should keep watching the two, for what are felicitous beginnings usually end differently. As a talkative patient explains:

> Ha! What you're seeing is their good side. Pearl's always swishing in here like she's Miss Happy-go-Lucky. Boy, does she love the news. She's always coming up to me and asking me how Marie's doing and . . . well, she's nice enough about it. I can't complain. It's better than most of them. I just tell her straight, like "Marie's fine," or "Marie's down," or something. You know what I mean? But wait . . . wait a bit and all hell breaks loose. You'll see. Just watch some time.

The comment prompts me to watch and listen closely. In time, I begin to discern the pattern cited earlier. Following an initial, cheerful greeting, Pearl typically asks Marie whether she has eaten all the food she has been offered that day and if Marie is being sociable. Regardless of the state of Marie's initial receptivity, a series of strong opinions is forthcoming. Following Pearl's inquiry about

Marie's eating regimen, Marie snidely responds that she, Marie, has always seen to the nutrition of her own family and, as for herself, is doing just fine under the circumstances. Then, again snidely, Marie wonders aloud whether Pearl is doing equally well for herself and her family. It is Marie's habit to turn Pearl's seemingly innocent questions into a commentary on Pearl's domestic habits, about which Pearl is very touchy. This usually is the start of an argument.

Pearl and Marie have different opinions of what "sets things off" whenever they get together. Pearl explains that what starts out as a very nice visit usually turns into a brawl because her mother soon "jabs" her about the way she takes care of her home:

> *It's always the same. I try my best to be cheerful. Really, I come here with the best of intentions. It's very important that Mother eat all her food. She's always been a very picky eater and I know if I don't keep track of her that she'll just not eat at all. So, you know, you try your best to not directly confront her, you know, kinda ask her about what she ate that day? But then, what do you know, she's jabbing me about what I feed Mike [her husband] and how she fed us better when we were kids. That's how she sets me off. She really knows how to twist the knife.*

Marie's interpretation is different. What Pearl defines as her mother's constant invidious comparisons, Marie says is an attempt to get Pearl to pay more attention to her own family and be less concerned with how Marie is doing. Marie explains how she never has felt Pearl was capable of taking care of herself, let alone a family:

> *You see, she's [Pearl] a worry to me. She's always been a worry to me, ever since she was little. She was always the kind of person that, if you don't prepare it for them, they starve. It's a constant worry. [Lengthy examples are presented.] She comes in here and tries to turn the tables on me . . . like I'm not eating well or something and, really, it's her that's probably not eating right. And I want to know! So I just ask her, point blank. Well . . . she doesn't like that. Oh . . . it's just a mother and a daughter having a friendly squabble.*

Few of those who have observed the squabbles call them friendly. To others, the squabbles are hostile, bitter, vulgar, and emotional. Some even describe the hostility as coming in stages! First are the recriminations. Marie touts her own history of domestic responsibility in comparison with Pearl's, which Pearl in turn lambasts as lies and wishful thinking. Then follows a stage of yelling about the relative truthfulness of claims concerning their treatment of their husbands, the cleanliness of their homes, and the care of their children. This leads to a stage of bitter recollection, focused on domestic crises each claims the other did nothing to resolve. This typically progresses to a fourth stage of vulgar character assassination. Finally, one of them sobs loudly, accusing her counterpart of not caring "a goddamn about me." Pearl and Marie rarely leave each other's company on good terms.

Family members report that Pearl and Marie always have had a stormy relationship. Several recount in broad detail the very stages others witness on a weekly basis. Pearl's sister even jokes about it:

> Those two. Have they been at it again? [I describe a recent visit.] So what's new? Tell me. Those two are like a broken record. And they can get pretty foul sometimes. Have you noticed any of that? Marie'll call her a selfish bitch and Pearl'll shoot right back that Mother's always been a jealous witch. Yeah, it gets that bad. Right? And then one of them starts to cry? Right? The trick is to wait for one of them to cry. Then you know it's over. Like her feelings have been hurt. [Sarcastically] Poor thing. Christ! Will it ever end? They were like that at home. Growing up wasn't very pleasant with those two around. Believe me. People don't change. What you're seeing is what Karen [a sister] and I heard all the time when we were kids. But, you know, it's what keeps 'em going. All that shit each of them brings up all the time. . . . It's tight. If it was me, I'd never come back.

Thus the sister suggests Pearl and Marie's visitations can be understood as part of a long history of interpersonal acrimony, emotional expressiveness, and resilient bonding. Pearl's sister notes that the two keep conjuring up old hostilities, but are nonetheless "tight."

Because of the acrimony, the facility's social worker persuades Pearl to participate in the support group she has organized for family members. The social worker thinks Pearl can benefit from sessions stressing effective visitation. Herb had been persuaded to attend the same sessions; in his case, it was believed there was a need to learn how to express, not control, feelings. The social worker explains that successful intervention has to strike a proper balance between the expression and control of emotions. Pearl, she points out, is a clear case of a family member who has to get a hold of herself and learn to let bygones be bygones.

There are clear and curious differences of opinion about whether the sessions enhance visitation. Pearl first states that the sessions make her more aware of how she and her mother set each other off, something she then adds she knows anyway. But then Pearl states that she attends the sessions as a favor to the social worker, whom she admires. As Pearl explains, "I've got the time anyway; so why not make her [the social worker] happy?" The social worker, too, is of mixed opinion about Pearl's response. At one point, the social worker describes what she sees as "real improvement" in Pearl's relations with her mother. Later, she sighs exasperatedly, "Those two? They'll always be like that," adding that, in such cases, what the support group and effective visitation provide is a forum for venting feelings, which helps in its own right, but does not really change situations that much.

Taken together, the remarks and occurrences draw attention to the place of life history in families' relations. Families bring interpersonal traditions to their encounters in nursing homes. Pearl's visits vividly depict what is carried forward in life. Like others, Pearl is not just a visitor nor Marie just a patient. They have been daughter and mother to each other and continue to be in their fashion. Tradition informs their current ties and related troubles. Visitation is a link in a more or less continuous chain of episodes in the history of people's lives, Pearl's and Marie's included.

The social worker's effort on behalf of effective visitation, well meant as it is, works at cross purposes with some patients' and families' ties and traditions. In theory, visits can be "treated" to make them more cordial and mutually beneficial. The idea of effective visitation assumes that. But this ignores the fact that social histories of cordiality, charity, hostility, volatility, and the like are simultaneously at work. Families are interlopers whose visits are always in some sense embedded in their pasts, producing stories too diverse to be easily contained by the relatively homogeneous aims of the present.

Implications for the Professional Caregiver

Each story in this chapter presents a family member as an interloper in the affairs of the nursing home to show the interpersonal and biographical complexity of the real world linking frail elderly and their families. Eula infringes on the unit's "bed-and-body" work. Maxine ostensibly makes an appearance when it suits her, when the presumed glamor of her other commitments does not keep her from seeing her father. This grates on the staff's sensibilities. Herb allegedly refuses to acknowledge and confront his feelings, fussing instead about the details of his mother's daily living. When Pearl visits her mother, there are almost certain to be arguments and acrimony, which does not sit right with many staff members and residents, because it is often at odds with the decorum of the environs. The complications and differences have implications for the service provider.

HOMOGENIZATION

Because the nursing home is a formal organization, there is an institutional tendency toward a homogenization of participants into official role players—into family members, patients, residents, and staff. This dissolves personal and interpersonal ties and traditions into organizational categories, also noted in relation to the community. While Eula's and Pearl's relations with their institutionalized family members contrast, they are nonetheless approached as visitors. While by her own reckoning, Maxine has a unique lifelong relationship of love and mutual support with her father, this is overlooked by the staff, who are alert to signs of not caring. While Herb has always just let feelings fall into place and never attempted to manage them, the social worker's professional, therapeutic concern with feelings finds Herb's approach lacking, if not unrealistic.

But, in the real world, sociability is not just a matter of visiting. In the nursing home, contacts between frail elderly and their families are interpersonal encounters between spouses, adult children and parents, and professional caregivers, among others, who bring with them manifold agendas and categories for interpreting one another's actions.

While there is a tendency to homogenize, which is an organization's way of rationalizing its activities, the organization produces diverse, but inherent troubles because official roles come into conflict with biographical particulars. Because of this, no nursing home can hope to make visits simply pleasant and personally profitable, even while fine efforts may be mounted on behalf of good family relations. While, in theory, a family member might be taught active listening or effective visitation, in practice what is learned is mediated by particular historical and social ties. Stories make the impasse evident.

THE LIMIT OF PROGRAM EFFECTIVENESS

The lesson to be learned from recognizing the tension between interpersonal ties and traditions on the one side, and organizational rhythms and sentiments on the other, is that families will always present a certain measure of troubles for nursing homes, just as outsiders "strangely" affect organizations in general. The assessment of program effectiveness might take this effect into account, lest the best laid plans of professional workers be unduly blamed for the by-products of inexorable organizational realities. As far as quality assurance is concerned, it is one thing to run a tight ship; it is quite another to attempt the impossible.

CHAPTER 7

Conceptualizing Intervention in the Real World

Consideration of frail elderly and their families in the real world began with a story about John, Phoebe, Miss Hanson, their friends, associates, and enemies. Details of the characters' lives were presented to show how ties, traditions, and troubles diversified the meaning of shared experiences. Other stories extended the argument well beyond the assumptions of rational planning, linear modeling, and single-perspective quality assessment. What seemed in theory to be straightforward and clean-cut, in practice engaged social and cultural complications.

In the process, implications for the professional caregiver were discussed. The linear view of adjustment, for example, did not provide a framework for stories that portray responses to the care experience as a multidimensional, multiperspectival configuration of adaptations. A comparison of themes and plots convoluted time beyond the usual developmental view. Whether the concern was community living, home care, institutionalization, or institutional life, the professional caregiver in the real world risked being ineffective when he or she formulated an approach without taking account of diversity and maintaining a healthy tolerance for the inconclusiveness, emergent meanings, unpredictability, and inventiveness of interpersonal encounters.

Establishing a Conceptual Space
Between Theory and Practice

In presenting stories, taking stock of contrasting theoretical formulations, and considering implications for the professional caregiver, the aim is to establish a space between theory and practice for conceptualizing intervention in the real world. In the process, a language is developed for addressing the real world in its own terms.

Rather than privileging theory and forming judgments about how theory is confounded by practice, how the real world poorly represents the ideal, or offering suggestions for how practice might better approximate theory, theory is made to take the stand, as it were. While this is standard procedure in science, the world of professional activity tends to reverse the relationship. Theory gains such administrative momentum as to become untestable, surviving not because it is supported by the facts of the real world, but because it validates professionalism. As theory gets bound up with organizational priorities, individual professional insight and discretion are constrained by job requirements, institutionalized goals, and official treatment philosophies.

Story opens a conceptual space to provide a basis for addressing in its own terms the problems that the real world poses for theory. Story permits plot development, that is, the presentation of the personal complications of lines of experience. The question of institutionalization, for example, is not addressed in terms of variables such as social support or felt burden, but considered according to the ways these factors are meaningfully articulated in particular cases. Stories not only show variation, but, more importantly, the qualitatively distinct forms these factors take in everyday life.

Story also permits multiperspectival character development. Both the character of John's behavior, and John as a character, differ according to John, Phoebe, and Miss Hanson. Maxine is one character in the version of her story she forms around her historical ties with her father and a vastly different character in the version floor staff share about her "flaunting" encounters with them. While story does not permit one to conclude which version is correct or more authentic, it does provide a vocabulary by which to appreciate and communicate differences.

The acknowledgement of a space between theory and practice is evident in the daily affairs of professional workers. Commonplace references to the "art" of professional activity are telling in this regard. Physicians speak of doctoring as going beyond theory, "booklearning," or received wisdom, among other references to an untaught domain of medical knowledge. They call the domain the "art of medicine." The art of medicine reaches into the categorical and working spaces of the real world to fit its complications and understandings with what is contrastingly called the "science of medicine." Likewise, nurses contrast nursing science with the art of nursing, social workers distinguish social work theory from social work practice, and other therapists and semiprofessional workers contrast what is called theory with what is relevant in the real world.

Harold Garfinkel (1967), a pioneer in the empirical study of this "art," has the domain in mind when he writes of the "artfulness" of everyday life. He means something akin to what the professional worker refers to when he or she speaks of the art of medicine, nursing, social service, and so on. Artfulness pertains to the practical reasoning engaged in sorting through experience and assigning meaning to its objects and events. The idea of story highlights the diverse, more or less complete, end-products—the plots and themes—of this artfulness.

Beyond Story

The mosaic of care is not just a collection of stories. Maxine's story takes on its meaning against larger questions and understandings, such as conceptions of satisfactory visitation and ideas about the interpersonal relations of families. Wilma's story of making a new home in the facility where she resides gains a larger significance in the context of the common vision of institutional living as the opposite of home. Mary's story teaches that figuring when "it's time" is not simply a matter of reaching the limits of one's tolerance in relation to the burden of care, but involves matching one's stresses and strains against what others view as filial responsibility.

The idea of a continuum of care provides one of the broadest and most publicly recognized contexts for stories. Indeed, one might have figured that the organization of chapters in this book reflects the continuum, from home care to institutional living. Against the background of stories, however, the continuum has many notable exceptions. Wilma learns to turn an institution into a home, resisting the tendency to impose hospital-like environs on personal space. Sophie, in occasionally suffering the pain of longing for home, shows that the past differentially enters separate moods of the present. In one mood, Sophie's past makes the present reasonable; in another mood, the past casts a sorrowful shadow on her current situation. As a family member, Ginny cannot "adjust" by forgetting the past, that is, putting it behind her. The past she has been told to forget makes meaningful much of what she still loves and cherishes. The fiercely independent Ben not only avoids attempts to link his life with service notions about the natural history of frailty, but altogether resists the imposition of the very idea of care. Ben has as little use for current intervention as he has use for a future defined in its terms.

The idea of a mosaic of care takes the designated realities of frail elderly and families to heart. It accepts the "family" that a single caregiver like Bea has with her close friends. For her, it is an important ingredient of her caregiving experience, as real in her sentiments as legal or biological kin (Gubrium & Holstein, 1990). "Family" is a way Bea assigns meaning to intimate relations. As such, Bea diversifies the definition of family caregiving well beyond common considerations of family support and responsibility. The mosaic of care takes seriously what frail elderly and their families define as real, resisting preexisting definitions. Not only does the mosaic of care delineate frailty and caregiving, but it takes account of how those whose lives are served align frailty and care and how they assign them meaning.

Stories, moreover, are more than just tales. They are about experiences, about ties, traditions, and troubles. In the real world, trouble relates to what people currently mean and have meant to each other. Story is a means of making the links between the three visible, a way of showing how the diverse facts of individual lives, while separate and distinct, nonetheless can be understood generally.

At the same time, it is important to take account of certain delimited domains of meaning in the real world as contexts for understanding life themes. For example, while the troubles of frail elderly and their families can be appreciated by means of stories of troubles, ties and traditions, there are places and circumstances in which stories are similarly thematized. As a delimited place, the nursing home provides a local culture for interpreting ties, traditions, and troubles, an important theme of which is dementia. Likewise, family members who participate in support groups for the caregivers of Alzheimer's disease victims learn that their ties with victims are likely to be invidiously compared with local exemplars of caregiving and evaluated in relation to notions of personal adjustment prevalent in the groups.

Conceptualizing intervention in the real world goes beyond story into order to compare and address the significance of differences, not to ultimately turn away from stories altogether. Maintaining a focus on story is a way of keeping from going too far beyond the real world of frailty, care, and caregiving. This produces a considerable conceptual tension because the generalizing thrust of theory tends to veer away from the particularizing quality of story. But it is a tension worth tolerating, better yet, sustaining, lest the real world be kept at arms distance from theory.

Subjective Relevance

It is easy to assume that one knows what people mean from listening objectively to what they say, and also to assume that what people do before one's very own eyes is something that has concretely happened. Stories inform us that both assumptions are dubious.

As far as knowing what people mean by what they say, take Harry's or Lucy's story. Both are ardent home caregivers for an elderly spouse. Harry cares for his disabled wife in their small apartment and, to the extent he can, takes her along with him in his car as he goes about his business. Some say that Lucy cares for a vegetative husband like a martyr, beyond what any mere mortal could do or bear in the circumstance. Others believe she is denying the fact that it is time to place him in a nursing home.

On various occasions, both are either asked, or freely speak, about the stresses and strains associated with home care. Harry remarks more than once that it is difficult to keep lifting Ruth in and out of the car. He is elderly himself and does not have the strength he once did. In his apartment, he speaks of all the details he has to attend to as he goes about his day managing the household. Yes, home care is a "bitch," as he sometimes remarks, and so is old age. And yes, too, there is much strain associated with caring for Ruth in her condition. "It's hell to grow old!" he asserts as he describes the difficulty of being Ruth's legs, arms, and, lately, her mind.

It is evident that Lucy, while a martyr to some and a denier to others, is aware of the work "it" all entails, meaning taking care of Melvin, her husband. As she goes about her household chores, she remarks both directly and in passing that it sometimes hurts her back to lift and turn Mel. She mentions how she wishes he could tell her what he needs or how he feels. Nonetheless, as she points out, she can tell in her own way what is on his mind and his emotional state by the little hints she detects in his eyes and from other bodily signs. Lucy, too, is never loathe to speak about how "stressed out," as she puts it, the caregiver can get, warning anyone who contemplates home care that it "ain't no picnic."

From these remarks it might be guessed, especially if one had the linear reasoning of the care equation in mind, that both are experiencing considerable strain in home care, both recognize it in their own ways, and one of them, Lucy in particular, is denying caregiving's impact on the caregiver. From this, one might readily conclude that both were candidates for "burn out," a "breakdown," or the serious consideration of care alternatives. According to the care equation, both Harry and Lucy are ripe for entertaining nursing home placement. In fact, when they are actually assessed on caregiver questionnaires, many of whose items serve to evaluate the felt burden of care, they are found to be highly stressed.

Yet in relation to their stories, in which the native categories and connections of experience are conveyed, their remarks and responses take on different meanings. In the context of his story, Harry's stress is the least he can put up with for his Ruth. For Harry, it is the mere physical side of care that proves stressful. The rest—all that he could do for his Ruth—is different. Different is Harry's life's work: caring for Ruth and being devoted to her as a loving husband. Stress, strain, or the burden of care, whatever it is called, has nothing to do with that commitment, according to Harry. In the context of Lucy's story, the question of institutionalization is linked to loss of companionship. The burden of care is what she, in effect, pays for keeping her lifelong friend at her side. Nursing home placement would be infinitely more painful than the stress of home care. It would mean being alone and lonely, "with no one around, no one to talk to, no one to hear me harp on everything," she surmises.

In separating parts of experience from other parts, one can easily assign them meanings of one's own choosing, not necessarily those conferred by their subjects. This is readily, and rather crudely, done in applying standardized modes of inquiry such as question-naires and other fixed assessment devices. Indeed, the aim to stan-dardize questions and responses in its own right works against story, for story tolerates complexity, inconclusiveness, and diversity in the meaning of words and deeds.

The same criticism applies to the interpretation of what one sees people do. The issue is highlighted in Bea's story. She is a single caregiver. She has no formal family of her own and therefore is believed to be the "logical" one to care for an elderly mother. But listening to Bea interpret her presumed lack of competing familial ties shows that she is being forced to rip herself away from those she loves and cares about as family. Bea's close friends, companions, and confidants are family. Putting into effect her presumed obligation to care for her mother full-time, she feels like she has given up on her "family." She is not as much stressed by home care as she is bereft of old and deeply meaningful ties.

Knowing what people mean by what they say and seeing what they are doing requires a commitment to understanding sub-jective relevance. The professional worker who aims to understand the real world must orient to its subjects' interpretations, in partic-ular, how interpretations are organized and the circumstances in which they are set forth. This provides a basis for discovering meanings that may be at odds with theory. The subject is not predefined as the service-defined client, but one whose story is told according to native understandings, varying according to its authors or storytellers.

The idea of version takes subjective relevance to mean that any one subject's or individual's version is not the whole story. Subjective relevance is neither mentalistic or individualistic, but perspectival. The subject of a story is not alone in defining its relevance. Indeed, subjective relevance extends to the professional worker's service-oriented version. More importantly, though, it does not selectively exclude the versions of frail elderly, their families, and significant others. In the context of subjective relevance, the profes-sional worker's account is one version, not the whole story, just as the person whom the story is about has a version of his or her story, again not the whole story. The point is that the commitment to subjective relevance does not seek some absolute truth in lives, but provides a guideline for revealing and appreciating the meanings that living can have.

Dynamic Construction

In the literary world, it is said that the best stories are written out of their authors' experiences. The commitment to subjective relevance borrows from this, while dynamically broadening authorship. The stories presented earlier not only cast experiences according to their expressed points of view, but their meanings are constructed according to their authors' related ties, traditions, and sense of troubles.

John's story, for one, tells of how events can be construed. John assembles events as a plan to "get back at the old bags." He tells of how he has been bothered for too long and has to get even. Taking advantage of the official designation of public space, he saunters down a hall and invades what is otherwise exclusively claimed. Phoebe constructs an entirely different version of events. To Phoebe and her friends, the bathroom incident is one more outrage from a man who is insufferably lewd and demented. Confronting Miss Hanson are diverse constructions. She cannot sort events from their versions.

But versions are not fixed constructs. They develop and change over time. In the real world, authorship is dynamic. Wilma's story is not just about institutional living. What she conveys about her experiences in living in a nursing home is a developing account. Her version of what is happening changes along with its events. At first her story reflects what some, like Goffman, describe as the self-mortification of the total institution. Wilma has lost her home and the way of life she has known. She denigrates her individuality and has become just another patient—a faceless, virtually lifeless, relatively well-cared-for prop in a hospital-like setting. In time we find that the setting gains a new significance for her. Her story changes to become one about daily resistance to invasions of privacy and infringements on personhood.

Mary's story, too, changes as she learns from other members in her support group about how to figure when "it's time" to seek nursing home placement. She discovers that there are different ways to construe the labors of home care and the resulting conflicting sentiments of caring for a degenerating loved one with a husband in the background. Like other authors who live in their own stories, Mary thematizes and plots her story in the very process of its construction. In the proceedings of her support group, Mary finds that versions are transformed into other versions. In this sense, stories are inconclusive, flowing with the enduring interpretation of the characters who author them.

The attempt to get to the bottom of stories confronts the attempt itself. Miss Hanson finds, for example, that as she tries to "get the story" of what happened in the bathroom incident, she becomes involved with its characters, becoming one herself. The involvement itself shapes varied versions. Ginny's story changes as she keeps looking back on her husband's nursing home placement, refiguring the meaning of institutionalization.

An appreciation of the dynamic construction of stories in the real world requires a tolerance for shifts in interpretation. It requires intervention attuned to how frail elderly and their families put together the meaning of their lives *as they experience them*. This is not easy because it moves in a direction opposite to closure. The dynamic under consideration here is different from linear change; it refers to the continuous construction of experience.

Embeddedness

Dynamic as it is, the construction of experience is not haphazard. While Wilma, for one, changes her mind about what life can be in the nursing home, she does not construct it willy nilly. She attends to the prevailing life themes in such a facility, organized as polarities, such as the opposition of home and hospital. While Wilma authors her story, she constructs it in the cultural context of the nursing home. Just as lived stories flow with experience and their versions link ties, traditions, and troubles, so their meanings are circumscribed by the existing understandings of place and time.

In a caregiver support group where the prevailing understanding is that the caregiver proceeds expeditiously to recognize that the personal needs of the caregiver are just as important as the needs of the care receiver, many stories are told about participants who dwell on the care receiver and deny reality. In a support group whose local culture is comprised of exemplars of total devotion and continued concern for cure and medical breakthrough, relatively few stories of denial are conveyed. In such a support group, a caregiver whose tie with the care receiver are founded on a tradition of long-term resentment stands to be considered callous and irresponsible when he or she raises the issue of institutionalization. In a support group tightly managed by facilitators and veteran participants who hold a decidedly linear view of caregiver adjustment, the caregiver whose ties with the care receiver are presented in terms of total filial responsibility risks being labeled as "denying" when the question of institutionalization is discussed.

The professional worker who takes subjective relevance into account and tolerates diversity in the construction of accounts risks seeing stories as individually idiosyncratic unless he or she considers the local cultural context in which stories are embedded. To take local culture into account is to realize, for example, that the troubles of adjustment being experienced by a devoted caregiver in a linearly oriented support group are, to some extent, the personal articulation of a group sentiment. Not taking local culture into account easily leads to the conclusion that the caregiver's troubles are completely his or her own.

Story as Attitude and Commitment

Orienting to a space between theory and practice offers a working attitude. Story takes priority over formal assessment. Version takes precedence over fact. The idea, of course, is that assessment and fact derive meaning in relation to understandings, experience, and social relations. Put into practice, story makes visible and serious what otherwise are dismissed as professional anecdotes, if not annoyances.

As a working attitude, story is a moral commitment. It adheres to the priority of the meanings and the significance of circumstance in the lives of all involved in caregiving, as diverse and multifaceted as the lives are. The commitment stands to reveal and enhance an appreciation of the many voices that constitute and reconstruct the lives of frail elderly and their families. The stories in this book tell as much.

Appendix—Methodology

*W*hile the research projects from which the stories in this book are taken vary in their focus, all are based on narrative material. From the beginning, 1969, not only behavior and patterns of inter-action are examined, but especially the *meaning* of conduct, inter-personal relations, and issues of living. If anything prominent can be said to have been thematic over the years, it is not a particular data-gathering technique, research design, or method for processing information, but rather an orientation to understanding.

Theory as Method

Lest readers be frustrated by the lack of a central concern with technique in a discussion of methodology, I should point out that it is important to think, in the first and final analysis, of theory as being one's primary method. What techniques do, which will be described shortly, is to process information or data. While this facilitates the formal organization of facts, it does not interpret them. Interpretation comes from an orientation to everyday life, which involves assumptions about the relation of individuals to their circumstances, the shape and strength of ties between people, and the place of tradition in their lives, among a host of other conceptual matters. In data-gathering, it does make a difference whether, say, one takes circumstance to be paramount in personal decision making or, in reverse order, emphasizes the shaping of circumstance by decision making. The former presents stories as products of life settings or narrative contexts; the latter highlights the influence persons' actions and interactions have on their circumstances.

It is perhaps an occupational hazard of social theorists that they are inclined to integrate into coherent systems the tensions between competing or contradictory concepts. The concepts of action and context, for example, are somewhat at odds. One emphasizes the voluntary activity of persons while the other underscores the effect of surroundings in shaping that activity. One way of linking them is to define one concept in terms of the other. It might be argued that surroundings such as communities and cultures are the historical and continuing by-products of personal and interpersonal actions.

My own feeling about the inclination is that, while it may be intellectually satisfying, it constrains the understanding of everyday life. The intellectual neatness produced by a coherent system of concepts shortchanges the loose ends, contradictions, multiple points of view, and complex interests—the many stories and versions—of the real world. My instinct is to tolerate the tension between analytic concepts, in the same way that those studied tolerate them in their own fashion because they live in the real world. It is a position against theoretical integration.

The method of analysis I have chosen in presenting the stories and versions of this book, combines two different kinds of concept. One kind gives a place to the voices of diverse parties. Story and version are a means of hearing, as it were, the different ways meaning can be attached to events, problems of living in particular. From a different kind of concept—including ties and traditions—the sense is that, while these voices are conveyed by their spokespersons, they are articulated in relation to who they now are and what they have been to each other. The emphasis also comes in the concept of life themes and localized understandings.

The Field Sites

The stories come from many field sites. A variety of methods were applied at the sites, from participant observation and the use of key informants to formal interviews and content analysis.

URBAN NEIGHBORHOODS

Some of the stories were of inhabitants of working-class and middle-class neighborhoods located in a large Midwestern, industrial city (Gubrium, 1973). The target sample was originally used to study the effect of old people's residential environments on their overall life satisfaction. Life in different kinds of noninstitutional housing was compared: single-family homes, apartments, single-room occupancy hotels, and public housing for seniors. Care was taken to separate out the effects of health, solvency, and social support. Some of the questions put to respondents were closed-ended, such as how strongly they agreed or disagreed that daily life is becoming difficult. Other questions were open-ended and requested them to explain or convey their opinions and feelings about specific concerns.

The open-ended questions in particular prompted respondents to tell stories. It was not unusual for the interviews to become extended conversations. In fact, it often was difficult to launch into a formal interview before time was taken to get acquainted and, in the process, hear and share stories. These were, after all, not just respondents, but people who lived and expected to continue participating in their worlds. It was out of these worlds that both formal interview responses and stories were conveyed, which I quickly learned gave shape and meaning—a vibrant context—to individual remarks.

Many stories were enriched by reports of what others thought. For example, an 86-year-old widow who lived alone in what was believed to be an unsafe neighborhood told the story of how she was "making it" on her own. She felt that her son, who lived in a distant suburb, viewed her circumstances differently. The widow presented both her own story and a version of it. In the process, I became intrigued by how service providers viewed the various lives they dealt with in the same neighborhoods, to present their own sundry stories.

MURRAY MANOR

In 1973, I formally entered a field site in another city to study it ethnographically (Gubrium, 1975). This was a nursing home I called "Murray Manor." The Manor had the reputation of being one of the finest facilities in the area. It was church-related and, at that time, housed 130 patients and residents on three floors. Residents were housed on the first floor, were ambulatory, and officially only required personal care. Patients made up the remainder and had rooms on the other floors. Two-thirds of the patients and residents paid for their care privately; others were supported by Medicaid.

Over the years, I have used a number of concepts to analyze the diversity of their experiences, especially as it presents itself in caregiving. An early one I applied to interpret the Murray Manor data was the idea that an organization such as a nursing home literally contains different *worlds* of care. The argument was that, in practice, a single formal organization can be several organizations for those playing various roles within it. I showed how members of the Manor's separate worlds—top (administrative) staff, floor staff, and clientele—assigned different and often contradictory meanings to the same conditions and events. This was the facility where John's story and its many versions were encountered.

OTHER NURSING HOMES

The nursing home research was extended to four other facilities in the same city (Gubrium, 1980a, 1980b). One was Brawley, a home specializing in the care of blind elderly. Two of the three others were for-profit facilities. The fourth was church-related.

The focus of analysis shifted from the differential worlds of care to the question of how contrasting professional languages of service workers were integrated into coherent portrayals of caregiving and clinical intervention. It was evident that in their professional or semi-professional capacities, physicians spoke differently from nurses about care, social workers differently from nurses, and therapists differently from activity workers. I was concerned with how the differences were resolved to present coherent stories about patient care for records and for regulating and funding agencies. Also of concern was the way external accountability was taken into consideration by staff members in formulating care plans.

WILSHIRE HOSPITAL

This growing interest led to research on the effects of audience on the communication of treatment and recovery. The site for this study was a physical rehabilitation hospital called "Wilshire" (Gubrium & Buckholdt, 1982), where fieldwork was conducted in 1979-80. The hospital treated the physical dysfunctions associated with brain trauma, stroke, spinal cord injury, amputation, and hip fracture. Most patients were elderly. The average length of stay was four to six weeks. The data were interpreted to show that what was said about treatment, and how progress was communicated, depended significantly on whether the audience was the patient, the family, or outside agents such as insurance companies.

Wilshire's clinical staff dealt with family members in a number of ways. Of particular interest were family conferences and support groups for the caregivers of elderly who had suffered strokes or fractures from falls. These settings produced quite detailed and emotional stories articulating the ties and traditions surrounding the trouble that patients had been, and eventually would be, to family members and others.

THE ALZHEIMER'S DISEASE EXPERIENCE

In 1983, the focus of the fieldwork moved from formal treatment organizations to the homes of family caregivers for Alzheimer's disease victims. Of particular interest were caregiver support groups and local chapters of the Alzheimer's Disease and Related Disorders Association (Gubrium, 1986a). The research eventually centered on support group proceedings, at first on support groups in one city, then moving into groups in another city, and eventually to groups that had since formed in the first city. Discourse and narrative continued to be important data, this time fixed on the question of how the borders of the normal and pathological are communicatively sustained.

Again, troubles, ties, and traditions that figured in caregiving experiences were conveyed, the many versions of which sensitized me to specific life themes and the effects of local cultures. An important subsidiary question was how the caregiving folklore of individual support groups affected the contents of stories shared by participants.

NURSING HOME RESIDENTS' LIFE STORIES

The most recent research foray centers on the life stories of nursing home residents. It is a two-year longitudinal study supported by a grant from the National Institute on Aging (#R01-AG07985). The plan is to trace how life narratives change from the time the nursing home is entered into the many months afterward, in particular how the sense of life, self, home, and family are affected. The study is significant because it explores the nursing home experience in context of the life as a whole rather than viewing the experience in terms of immediate institutional conditions. While none of the stories presented in this book comes directly from this study, I mention it here to point out that the story not only has interpersonal versions sensitive to ties, traditions, and local cultures, but has an emergent context as well.

Taken together, the field sites offered stories of frail elderly and their families from a variety of backgrounds. Most were working class or middle class. To my knowledge, none was extremely wealthy nor were many from what is called the "underclass." Most of the elderly had worked all their lives and retired or, in the case of elderly women, had been homemakers. Some had become disabled early in life and "made do" the rest of it. Their ethnic origins were varied, too, and are apparent in some of the stories. Mainly, the elderly resided either in institutions or in urban neighborhoods; their families typically were suburban.

How the Stories Were Recorded

Stories were recorded in the process of both doing formal interviews and participant observation. During formal interviews, parts of stories were recorded by hand before, during, and immediately after I took leave of respondents. As near to exact testimony as possible eventually was written up for future reference. In some instances, only limited descriptions of lengthy tales and experiential details could be noted.

During participant observation, the same process was followed when a tape recorder was not available or did not prove feasible to use. In the many conferences, meetings, support groups, and office interactions observed, participants were accustomed to note taking. Staff members often wrote during the proceedings, as did family members themselves. Casual visits to nursing home residents' and hospitalized patients' rooms, hallway observations, conversations at nurses' stations, and the like produced many and varied versions of events otherwise heard and communicated in other versions, at other times and in other places. Visits to family caregivers' homes provided additional narrative material.

Much of this has been edited for publication. Identifying references have been deleted or fictionalized. Redundant accounts have been shortened or excised, even those tape recorded. Elaborate details, often conveyed in the camaraderie of conversation, usually were not recorded by hand but, rather, simply specified or briefly described. The stories that appear in this book, then, are combinations of edited testimony and conversation, enriched by field observations.

References

Abel, Emily. 1989. "The ambiguities of social support: Adult daughters caring for frail elderly parents," Journal of Aging Studies 3:211–230.

Brody, Elaine. 1981. "Women in the middle and family help to older people," The Gerontologist 21:271–282.

Burnley, Cynthia S. 1987. "Caregiving: The impact of emotional support for single women," Journal of Aging Studies 1:253–264.

Donzelot, Jacques. 1979. The Policing of Families. New York: Pantheon.

Dovey, Kim. 1985. "Home and homelessness." In Irwin Altman & Carol M. Werner (eds.), Home Environments. New York: Plenum.

Emerson, Robert M. & Sheldon Messenger. 1977. "The micro-politics of trouble," Social Problems 25:121–134.

Evers, Helen. 1983. "Elderly women and disadvantage: Perceptions of daily life and support relationships." In Dorothy Jerrome (ed.), Ageing in Modern Society. London: Croom Helm.

Evers, Helen. 1985. "The frail elderly woman: Emergent questions in ageing and women's health." In Ellen Lewin & Virginia Olesen (eds.), Women, Health, and Healing. London: Tavistock.

Fischer, Lucy Rose, Leah Rogne & Nancy Eustis. 1990. "Care without commitment." In Jaber F. Gubrium & Andrea Sankar (eds.), The Home Care Experience. Newbury Park, CA: Sage.

Frankfather, Dwight. 1977. The Aged in the Community. New York: Praeger.

Frost, P.J., L.F. Moore, M.R. Louis, C.C. Lundberg & J. Martin. 1985. Organizational Culture. Beverly Hills, CA: Sage.

Garfinkel, Harold. 1967. Studies in Ethnomethodology. Englewood Cliffs, NJ: Prentice Hall.

Geertz, Clifford. 1983. Local Knowledge: Further Essays in Interpretive Anthropology. New York: Basic.

Glaser, Barney G. & Anselm L. Strauss. 1967. The Discovery of Grounded Theory. Chicago: Aldine.

Goffman, Erving. 1961b. "The moral career of the mental patient." In Erving Goffman, Asylums, New York: Doubleday.

Gubrium, Jaber F. 1973. The Myth of the Golden Years: A Socio-Environmental Theory of Aging. Springfield, IL: Charles C. Thomas, Publishers.

Gubrium, Jaber F. 1975. Living and Dying at Murray Manor. New York: St. Martin's.

Gubrium, Jaber F. 1980a. "Doing care plans in patient conferences," Social Science and Medicine 14A:659–667.

Gubrium, Jaber F. 1980b. "Patient exclusion in geriatric staffings," Sociological Quarterly 21:335–348.

Gubrium, Jaber F. 1986a. Oldtimers and Alzheimer's: The Descriptive Organization of Senility. Greenwich, CT: JAI Press.

Gubrium, Jaber F. 1986b. "The social preservation of mind: The Alzheimer's disease experience," Symbolic Interaction 6:37–51.

Gubrium, Jaber F. 1987b. "Structuring and destructuring the course of illness," Sociology of Health and Illness 3:1–24.

Gubrium, Jaber F. 1988a. Analyzing Field Reality. Newbury Park, CA: Sage.

Gubrium, Jaber F. 1988b. "Family responsibility and caregiving in the qualitative analysis of the Alzheimer's disease experience," Journal of Marriage and the Family 50:197–207.

Gubrium, Jaber F. 1988c. "Incommunicables and poetic documentation in the Alzheimer's disease experience," Semiotica 72:235–253.

Gubrium, Jaber F. 1989a. "Local cultures and service policy." In Jaber F. Gubrium & David Silverman (eds.), The Politics of Field Research: Sociology Beyond Enlightenment. London: Sage.

Gubrium, Jaber F. & David R. Buckholdt. 1977. Toward Maturity: The Social Processing of Human Development. San Francisco: Jossey-Bass.

Gubrium, Jaber F. & David R. Buckholdt. 1982. Describing Care: Image and Practice in Rehabilitation. Boston, MA: Oelgeschlager, Gunn & Hain.

Gubrium, Jaber F., David R. Buckholdt & Robert J. Lynott. 1989. "The descriptive tyranny of forms." In James A. Holstein & Gale Miller (eds.), Perspectives on Social Problems, vol. 1, Greenwich, CT: JAI Press.

Gubrium, Jaber F. & James A. Holstein. 1990. What is Family? Mountain View, CA: Mayfield Publishers.

Gubrium, Jaber F. & Robert J. Lynott. 1983. "Rethinking life satisfaction," Human Organization 42:30–38.

Gubrium, Jaber F. & Robert J. Lynott. 1985. "Family rhetoric as social order," Journal of Family Issues 6:129–152.

Gubrium, Jaber F. & Robert J. Lynott. 1987. "Measurement and the interpretation of burden in the Alzheimer's disease experience," Journal of Aging Studies 1:265–285.

Gubrium, Jaber F. & Andrea Sankar (eds.). 1990. The Home Care Experience: Ethnography and Policy. Newbury Park, CA: Sage.

Gwyther, Lisa P. & Linda K. George. 1986. "Introduction to symposium on caregivers for dementia patients: Complex determinants of well-being and burden," The Gerontologist 26:245–247.

Hilker, Mary Anne. 1987. "Families and supportive residential settings as long-term care options." In Timothy Brubaker (ed.), Aging, Health, and Family: Long-Term Care. Newbury Park, CA: Sage.

Hochschild, Arlie Russell. 1973. The Unexpected Community. Englewood Cliffs, NJ: Prentice-Hall.

Holstein, James. A. 1990. "Describing home care: Discourse and Image in involuntary commitment proceedings." In Jaber F. Gubrium & Andrea Sankar (eds.), The Home Care Experience: Ethnography and Policy. Newbury Park, CA: Sage.

Jerrome, Dorothy (ed.). 1983. Ageing in Modern Society: Contemporary Approaches. London: Croon Helm.

Johnson, Colleen L. & Leslie A. Grant. 1985. The Nursing Home in American Society. Baltimore: Johns Hopkins University Press.

Lasch, Christopher. 1979. Haven in a Heartless World. New York: Basic.

Lewis, Jane & Barbara Meredith. 1988. "Daughters caring for mothers: The experience of caring and its implications for professional helpers," Ageing and Society 8:1–21.

Manard, Barbara Bolling, Cary Steven Kart & Dirk W.L. van Gils. 1975. Old-Age Institutions. Lexington, MA: Lexington Books.

Mace, Nancy L. & Peter V. Rabins. 1981. The 36-Hour Day. Baltimore: Johns Hopkins University Press.

McPherson, Barry D. 1983. Aging as a Social Process. Toronto: Butterworth.

Mills, C. Wright. 1963. "The professional ideology of social pathologists." In C. Wright Mills, Power, Politics, and People. New York: Oxford University Press.

Morgan, David L. 1989. "Adjusting to widowhood: Do social networks really make it easier?" The Gerontologist 29:101–107.

Morycz, R.K. 1985. "Caregiving strain and the desire to institutionalize family members with Alzheimer's disease," Research on Aging 7:329–361.

Neugarten, Bernice L. 1974. "Age groups in American society and the rise of the young-old," Annals of the American Academy of Political and Social Science, Sept., 187–198.

Poster, Mark. 1978. Critical Theory of the Family. New York: Seabury.

Poulshock, S.W. & Gary T. Deimling. 1984. "Families caring for elders in residence: Issues in the measurement of burden," Journal of Gerontology 39:230–239.

Raffel, Stanley. 1979. Matters of Fact. London: Routledge & Kegan Paul.

Rubinstein, Robert. 1989a. "The home environments of older persons: A description of the psychosocial processes linking person to place," Journal of Gerontology 44:S45–53.

Rubinstein, Robert. 1989b. "Themes in the Meaning of Caregiving," Journal of Aging Studies 3:119–132.

Rubinstein, Robert. 1990. "Culture and disorder in the home care experience: The home as sickroom." In Jaber F. Gubrium & Andrea Sankar (eds.), The Home Care Experience. Newbury Park, CA: Sage.

Said, Edward W. 1978. Orientalism. New York: Random House.

Sankar, Andrea. 1986. "Out of the clinic into the home: Control and communication in patient-physician relations," Social Science and Medicine 22:973–982.

Sankar, Andrea. 1988. "The home as a site for teaching gerontology and geriatrics." In M. Lock & D. Gordon (eds.), Knowledge and Practice in Medicine. Holland: Reidel.

Schultz, Alfred. 1970. On Phenomenology and Social Relations. Chicago: University of Chicago Press.

Shield, Renee Rose. 1988. Uneasy Endings. Ithaca: Cornell University Press.

Simmel, Georg. 1950. The Sociology of Georg Simmel. New York: Free Press.

Spector, Malcolm & John Kitsuse. 1977. Constructing Social Problems. Menlo Park, CA: Cummings.

Sudnow, David (ed.). 1972. Studies in Social Interaction. New York: Free Press.

Waerness, Kari. 1984. "Caring as women's work in the welfare state." In Harriet Holfer (ed.), Patriarchy in a Welfare State. Oslo: Universitetsforlaget.

Wenger, G. Clare. 1987. "Dependence, interdependence, and reciprocity after eighty," Journal of Aging Studies 1:355–377.

Werner, Carol M., Irwin Altman, & Diane Oxley. 1985. "Temporal aspects of home: A transactional analysis." In Irwin Altman & Carol M. Werner (eds.), Home Environments. New York: Plenum.

Zarit, Steven H., Nancy K. Orr & Judy M. Zarit. 1985. The Hidden Victims of Alzheimer's Disease: Families Under Stress. New York: New York University Press.

Zarit, Steven H., K.E. Reever, & J. Bach-Peterson. 1980. "Relatives of the impaired elderly: Correlates of feeling of burden," The Gerontologist 20:649–655.

Index